OXFORD MEDICAL PUBLICATIONS

BRITISH PAEDIATRIC ASSOCIATION
MANUAL ON
INFECTIONS AND IMMUNIZATIONS IN CHILDREN

GW00503859

Steering and writing group:

Dr Angus Nicoll (co-editor) *Wellcome Lecturer in the Epidemiology of AIDS, London School of Hygiene & Tropical Medicine.*

Dr Peter Rudd (co-Editor) *Consultant Paediatrician, Children's Centre, Royal United Hospital, Bath.*

Professor Alex Campbell (**Convener**) *Professor of Child Health, Royal Aberdeen Children's Hospital.*

Professor John Forfar *Professor Emeritus of Child Life & Health, Edinburgh.*

Dr Susan Hall *Senior Lecturer in Paediatric Epidemiology, Institute of Child Health, London.*

Professor David Hull *Professor of Child Health, Nottingham University Hospital.*

Professor Roland Levinsky *Professor of Immunology, Institute of Child Health, London.*

Professor Richard Moxon *Professor of Paediatrics, John Radcliffe Hospital, Oxford.*

Professor Catherine Peckham *Professor of Paediatric Epidemiology, Institute of Child Health, London.*

Dr David Salisbury *Department of Health and Social Security.*

Dr Helen Zealley *Community Medicine Specialist, Astley Ainslie Hospital, Edinburgh.*

British Paediatric Association
Manual on
Infections and Immunizations
in Children

Edited by

Dr ANGUS NICOLL

Paediatrician and Epidemiologist
Department of Tropical Hygiene,
London School of Hygiene and Tropical Medicine

and

Dr PETER RUDD

Consultant Paediatrician
Royal United Hospital, Bath

Oxford   New York   Tokyo
OXFORD UNIVERSITY PRESS
1989

Oxford University Press, Walton Street, Oxford OX2 6DP

Oxford   New York   Toronto
Delhi   Bombay   Calcutta   Madras   Karachi
Petaling Jaya   Singapore   Hong Kong   Tokyo
Nairobi   Dar es Salaam   Cape Town
Melbourne   Auckland

and associated companies in
Berlin   Ibadan

Oxford is a trade mark of Oxford University Press

Published in the United States
by Oxford University Press, New York

British Library Cataloguing in Publication Data

British Paediatric Association manual on injections
and immunizations in children.
1. Children. Communicable diseases
I. Nicoll, Angus.   II. Rudd, Peter.
618.92'9
ISBN 0–19–261785–0

Library of Congress Cataloging in Publication Data

British Paediatric Association manual on infections
and immunizations in children.
Bibliography. Includes index.
1. Communicable diseases in children—Handbooks,
manuals, etc.   2. Immunization of children—Handbooks,
manuals, etc.   I. Nicoll, Angus.   II. Rudd, Peter.
III. British Paediatric Association.   IV. Title: Manual
on infections and immunizations in children.   [DNLM:
1. Communicable Diseases—in infancy & childhood—
handbooks.   2. Immunization—in infancy & childhood—
handbooks.   WC 39 B862]
RJ401.B75   1989   618.92'9   88–31255
ISBN 0–19–261785–0

Set by Latimer Trend & Company Limited

Printed and bound in Great Britain by
Biddles Ltd, Guildford and King's Lynn

Foreword

Mrs Edwina Currie, MP

Infectious diseases in children are common, they cause considerable and sometimes life-threatening illness, and promote much anxiety in parents. All those working with children need to have clear, up-to-date, and practical advice about infectious diseases and this book does this admirably. Many infectious diseases are preventable through immunization and it is vital that doctors, nurses and parents know the correct facts to promote immunization as much as possible. We must improve our performance in immunization and the advice contained in the book should help greatly.

As a Minister, with a commitment to prevention and health promotion, I warmly welcome the initiative of the British Paediatric Association in producing this publication.

Acknowledgements

We would like to thank all our paediatric collaborators who wrote sections of this book, particularly Professors Alex Campbell and John Forfar for their enthusiasm and support. Dr David Salisbury of the DHSS also sat on the committee to ensure close liaison with the JCVI. Other medical colleagues, manufacturers and authorities, too numerous to mention, contributed information or made valuable comments. We are grateful to them all. The Communicable Diseases Surveillance Centre (CDSC) London is the source of Figs 1, 3, 4, 5, and 6. C. V. Mosby and Company kindly gave permission for an illustration in *Infectious diseases for children* by S. Krugman and S. L. Katz to be used as a basis for Fig. 2. Mr Graham Doyal and the Vaccination and Immunization Committee of Nottingham Health Authority are the source of Figs 7, 8, and 9. The latter also kindly gave permission for us to use portions of its handbook as a starting point for large parts of the immunization section. The Malaria Reference Laboratory of the London School of Hygiene and Tropical Medicine gave advice on protection against malaria. Information on morbidity and mortality was taken from the published statistics of the Offices of Population Censuses and Surveys, the Health and Personal Social Services Department of the Northern Ireland Department, the Information Services Division of the Scottish Office, the General Register Offices of Scotland and Northern Ireland, the Weekly Returns Service of the Royal College of Practitioners, the British Paediatric Surveillance Unit, the Congenital Rubella Surveillance Programme, and was supplied by Dr Noel Gill of the CDSC. Professors John Forfar and June Lloyd carefully reviewed an early draft and made many helpful suggestions as to changes in the text. Finally we would like to acknowledge the efforts of Sheila Brizell, Jean Gaffin, Paul Dunn, and John Wilkins in the BPA office, in the preparation of the text.

Angus Nicoll
Peter Rudd

Preface

In the 1970s the publicity given to rare but serious brain damage apparently related to whooping cough vaccine overshadowed appreciation of the benefits of childhood immunization. The resulting loss of confidence (and fear of legal implications) among the doctors and nurses who carry out immunizing procedures further seriously undermined our national programme of immunization which already compared unfavourably with that of some other countries, notably the United States of America. British paediatricians have traditionally not been practically involved with immunization but have become increasingly concerned about the persisting morbidity and mortality from preventable infections such as measles. To reflect this concern the Council of the British Paediatric Association in 1982 initiated its Standing Committee on Immunization and Vaccination to explore ways in which paediatricians might help to promote immunization, develop mutually productive links with the DHSS Joint Committee on Vaccination and Immunization (JCVI) and provide advice and support to those doctors and nurses in the 'front line' of immunization practice.

It soon became apparent that the UK lacked a simple, yet reasonably comprehensive guide to infectious disease and immunization similar to the excellent *Red Book* produced by the American Academy of Pediatrics. This handbook is designed to fill that gap. It is not intended to replace or conflict with the official publications of the DHSS, and considerable care has been taken to ensure that the recommendations are consistent so that much confusion about immunization might be avoided in the future.

In collaboration with the BPA Immunology and Infectious Diseases Group a Steering Committee was formed and Drs Angus Nicoll and Peter Rudd were appointed editors. Under their guidance each contributor was asked to produce simple yet authoritative summaries of the important infections of childhood and practical guides to immunization that might answer most of the questions that arise every day in doctors' surgeries and clinics. While a book of this kind cannot be comprehensive enough to include all conditions encountered world-wide it must acknowledge the increasing opportunities that exist for families to travel abroad and become exposed to disorders not usually seen in the UK.

The first two sections immediately following this preface indicate that there is no room for complacency either about childhood morbidity and mortality, or about current levels of immunization uptake. Much remains to be done. We hope that this book will help.

How well we have succeeded will be for others to judge. Comments and suggestions will be valuable towards improving future editions as the book will remain useful only if it is updated regularly to take account of new developments in the rapidly changing scene of infectious disease.

A. G. M. Campbell
Convener, Standing Committee on Immunization and Vaccination

CONTENTS

Clinical Problems

Diseases

Immunization

Practical Immunization:
Questions and Answers

Travel Abroad

Appendices

Contents

Child mortality from infectious diseases in 1985   xvii

Child morbidity from infectious diseases in 1985   xviii

Immunization targets and uptake   xx

The British Paediatric Surveillance Unit   xxii

Introduction—how to use this book   xxiii

Clinical Problems

Infections in the new-born period and infancy   3

The child with respiratory infection   6

The child with a rash   13

The child with a fever   22

The child with urinary-tract infection   25

The child with vomiting and diarrhoea   28

The child with sexually transmitted disease   30

Congenital infections: management of important infections during pregnancy and the neonatal period   32

Diseases

AIDS/HIV   37

Chickenpox/Herpes zoster   43

Chlamydia trachomatis   46

Cholera   48

Cytomegalovirus   50

Diphtheria 52

Fifth disease 55

Gastrointestinal infections 57

Glandular fever 64

Gonococcal infections 66

Haemolytic uraemic syndrome 68

Haemophilus influenzae infection 70

Hand, foot, and mouth disease 73

Hepatitis A 75

Hepatitis B 77

Herpes simplex 80

Influenza 83

Kawasaki disease 85

Malaria 88

Measles 91

Meningococcal disease 95

Molluscum contagiosum 98

Mumps 99

Nits (*Pediculosis capitis*) 101

Pneumococcal infections 103

Poliomyelitis 105

Rabies 107

Respiratory syncytial virus (RSV) infection 109

Ringworm (Tinea) 111

Roseola infantum (exanthum subitum) 114

Rubella (German measles) 115

Scabies 119

Staphylococcal infections 121

Streptococcal infections 124

Tetanus 128

Threadworms 130

Thrush (candidiasis) 132

Toxocariasis (visceral larva migrans) 134

Toxoplasmosis 136

Tuberculosis (TB) 139

Typhoid fever 144

Warts and verrucae 146

Whooping cough (pertussis) 148

Yellow fever 152

The collection of specimens for the diagnosis of   153
infection

Immunization

General introduction 163

Vaccine handling 169

Preparing for immunization, medical prescriptions,   172
nurse immunizing, and parental consent

Parental counselling 174

Giving vaccines 176

Immunization reactions 182

Individual immunizations 187

Cholera 188

Diphtheria 190

Hepatitis B 192

Influenza 197

Measles/mumps/rubella (MMR) 200

Measles   205
Mumps   206
Pertussis (whooping cough)   207
Pneumococcus   211
Polio OPV   213
Polio IPV   216
Rubella   217
Tetanus   221
Tuberculosis   224
Typhoid   230
Yellow fever   232
Immunoglobulins given to children   234

Practical Immunization: Questions and Answers

Practical immunization: questions and answers   239
Immunization and protection of infants and children   256
    with specific problems

Travel Abroad

Travel abroad   265
The child travelling from abroad   279

Appendices

1 Notifiable diseases   284
2 Anti-microbials   286
3 Exclusion periods   302
4 Immunization schedules   310
5 Sources of specialist advice   313

6 Current sources of supply of vaccines and other immunological products 316

7 Further reading 329

Glossary and abbreviations 332

Index 339

Child mortality from infectious diseases in the United Kingdom 1985

(International Classification of Disease Codes)

	0–1 yrs	1–4 yrs	5–10 yrs	Total
All infectious and parasitic disease (001–139)	120	77	42	239
Intestinal infectious disease (001–9)	28	4	3	35
Tuberculosis (010–18)	0	2	1	3
Other bacterial disease (020–41)	61	46	14	121
Diphtheria (032)	0	0	0	0
Whooping cough (033)	2	1	1	4
Meningococcal infection (036)	23	38	9	70
Septicaemia (038)	34	4	4	42
Viral disease (045–79)	26	22	20	68
Viral disease of the nervous system (045–9)	5	5	9	19
Acute polio (045)	0	0	0	0
Chickenpox (052)	3	1	5	9
Herpes simplex (054)	6	4	1	11
Measles (055)	3	5	2	10
Rubella (056)	0	0	0	0
Viral hepatitis (070)	0	1	4	5
Mumps (072)	0	0	0	0
Meningitis (320–2)	64	33	20	117
Acute bronchitis/bronchiolitis (466)	95	24	6	125
Pneumonia (480–6)	224	38	14	276
Infections specific to the perinatal period (771)	105	1	1	107
Sudden Infant Death Syndrome (798)[*]	1165	30	0	1195

[*]A number of these fatalities are associated with infections.

Child infectious disease morbidity

Notifications of disease

(in 1985; England and Wales only)

	All ages	0–4 yrs	5–14 yrs
Cholera	7	1	0
Typhoid	179	26	43
Dysentery	5335	1636	1449
Food poisoning (formally notified or ascertained by other means)	19 241	3182	1939
Jaundice	4382	167	962
Tuberculosis (all)	5857	168	263
Tuberculous meningitis	53	4	5
Diphtheria	4	0	1
Whooping cough	22 046	13 096	8105
Scarlet fever	6438	2073	3571
Acute meningitis	1531	689	245
meningococcal	549	253	103
pneumococcal	82	30	6
H. influenzae	206	193	2
Viral	323	85	72
Ophthalmia neonatorum	258	258	—
Tetanus	12	0	1
Measles	97 408	48 735	44 190
Polio (acute, paralytic and non-paralytic)	4	4	0
Malaria	1691	88	211

Diseases ascertained from special reporting schemes

A. National Congenital Rubella Surveillance Programme (NCRSP)

Congenital Rubella Syndrome (Great Britain): 20 cases reported in 1985.

B. Royal College of General Practitioners 'Spotter Practices' (mainly England and Wales), contains adult data for reference

	Average weekly rate per 100 000 pop. (1985)				
	0–4 yrs	5–14 yrs	15–44 yrs	45–64 yrs	65+ yrs
Chickenpox	57.82	37.05	4.67	0.51	0.13
Mumps	35.20	18.53	1.85	0.37	0.13
Rubella	24.83	9,68	0.69	0.09	0.07

C. British Paediatric surveillance Unit (British Isles), cases reported June 1986 to August 1987 (first year of operation)—includes some cases with onset before June 1986

Disease	Number of cases**
Acquired Immunodeficiency Syndrome (AIDS) in childhood	21
Haemolytic uraemic syndrome	74
Neonatal herpes	10
Sub-acute sclerosing panencephalitis (SSPE*)	26
Kawasaki disease	105

*   Primarily a complication of measles.
** Includes only cases followed up by investigations and confirmed as meeting case definition (as at 4.2.88).

Immunization targets

The decision to withold immunization should be taken only after serious consideration of the potential consequences for the individual child and the community.

WHO Expanded Programme on Immunization 1984

Realistic minimum targets

Polio Diphtheria Tetanus Pertussis	90 per cent of all children to have three doses by the second birthday
Measles/mumps/ rubella (MMR)	90 per cent of all children to be immunized by the second birthday; vaccine uptake should also be reviewed at school entry
Rubella	No girl should enter the child-bearing years susceptible to rubella

These targets are sufficient for satisfactory herd immunity for some diseases: measles, mumps, and pertussis. However, for individual protection the level of vaccine uptake should be exceeded. All health-care professionals should ensure that these targets are achieved for the children under their care. **Community paediatricians carry a particular responsibility in this respect in their own geographical area.**

Adapted from regional WHO targets for Europe 1984

National immunization uptake* (England only)

Diphtheria	85 per cent
Tetanus	85 per cent
Polio	85 per cent
Pertussis	68 per cent
Measles	71 per cent

* Children born 1984 completing primary immunization courses by 31.12.86.

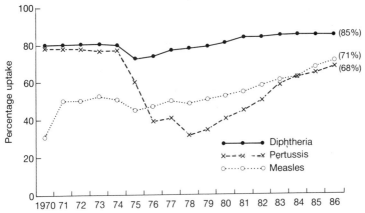

Fig. 1 Immunization uptake in England and Wales 1970–86.
Figures for the UK are similar, those for 1986 are only for England, and the figures for diptheria, tetanus, and polio are similar. Figures are computed for a year as the number of immunization courses (e.g. three Triples) completed by 31 December of that year for children who were born in the year preceding, divided by the number of live births in the latter year. For example, 1986 figures are all courses completed by 31.12.86 amongst children born in 1984, divided by the number of live births in 1984.

The British Paediatric Surveillance Unit (BPSU)

This unit was set up in 1986 on the initiative of the British Paediatric Association to facilitate the surveillance and study of rare childhood infections, infection-related, and other disorders by providing an 'active' case ascertainment facility. It is a joint venture of the British and Irish Paediatric Associations, the Communicable Disease Surveillance Centre, Communicable Diseases (Scotland) Unit, and the Department of Epidemiology of the Institute of Child Health, London.

A report card containing a list of conditions is sent monthly to all hospital consultant paediatricians in the UK and Eire. The reportable conditions involving infection in 1988 are:

- Acquired immunodeficiency syndrome (AIDS) in childhood;

- neonatal herpes;

- subacute sclerosing panencephalitis (SSPE);

- Reye's syndrome;

- haemolytic uraemic syndrome;

- Kawasaki disease;

- haemorraghic shock encephalopathy syndrome;

- (rheumatic fever, congenital rubella—one month only, retrospective surveys).

For further information contact the Medical Coordinator, BPSU, 5 St. Andrew's Place, London NW1 4LB. Telephone: 01–935 1866.

Introduction: how to use this book

This handbook is intended for all primary-care and hospital staff working with children: general practitioners, clinic doctors, paediatricians, health visitors, practice nurses, school nurses and clinic nurses, ward nurses, nursing students, junior doctors, and medical students. As a source of information on infectious diseases and immunization other child-care professionals, health administrators, and parents will also find parts of the text useful.

The text may be read through in its entirety but as a handbook it is designed as a source of information and guidance for the user with a specific problem. The organization of the book reflects this, with marginal flags to allow sections to be found with ease, and a number of appendices. A key to the marginal flags can be found on the first page of the list of Contents (p. ix). There is considerable cross-referencing and some repetition so that the reader does not have to skip around the book excessively.

The first section **Clinical problems** gives general guidance on the diagnosis and management of children with infection: respiratory illness, fever, rash, etc. When a variety of organisms may be the cause (e.g. otitis media) some guidelines on treatment are provided in these pages. However, if a more specific diagnosis is possible the reader is referred on to the second section **Diseases** where the principal childhood infectious diseases are arranged alphabetically. Practical details are given for each concerning epidemiology (including mode of transmission and incubation periods), natural history, and management. Antibiotic dosage is given in Appendix 2 where this is appropriate. When diseases have only recently been recognized (examples are AIDS and Kawasaki disease) they are described in more detail; the same applies for newer immunizations (hepatitis B and MMR).

The third section concerns **Immunization** and describes in alphabetical order the vaccines available for children. This gives details for each vaccine of its efficacy, when it should be given, and the rare occasions when it should be withheld. Also in the section are given the essentials of immunization practice: vaccine handling, consent and medical prescription, and immunization reactions. A section **Practical immunization: questions and answers** covers the specific problems that arise in day-to-day immunization (for example, who gives consent when a child is a ward of court). Because of the increasing amount of international travel there is a section on **Travel abroad** concerning preparing for a trip, and including a sub-section on the management of an ill child recently arrived in the UK, **The child travelling from abroad**.

The appendices give lists of notifiable diseases, anti-microbials, exclusion periods, immunization schedules, sources of specialist advice, vaccine suppliers and further reading. There is also a glossary and index.

Inside the front and back covers is some information which may be required frequently (immunizations children should have by key ages, and an immunization checklist) or rapidly (managing anaphylaxis).

All the sections cover the activities of both primary and hospital care. A few of those involving very sick children (e.g. severe croup) or severe diseases (e.g. diphtheria) will only be applicable to hospital. Details of management of these conditions are given for the guidance of hospital staff and as information for community practitioners. This is evident from the text. The bulk of childhood infections are presently managed within the context of primary care and undoubtedly should continue to be so. Some cases of mild or moderate illness will benefit from hospital help or advice. The decision on whether to admit a child is rarely simple and this book does not attempt to provide hard and fast rules. Our experience as doctors working both in the community and hospital has convinced us of the importance of communication and discussion in the management of infectious disease. Likewise, a telephone consultation between hospital specialist and community practitioner can frequently resolve even quite difficult immunization problems.

The handbook details a single well-tried approach to most

problems of diagnosis and management of infection. However, there are often acceptable alternatives and we would not wish to imply that these should not be used.

Finally, we would like to welcome and encourage comments on this handbook so that second and subsequent editions may be improved.

April 1988

Angus Nicoll
Peter Rudd
British Paediatric Association

Clinical Problems

Infection in the new-born period and infancy

(Infancy is taken to include the first 12 months of life)

Infection presenting in the neonatal period (the first four weeks of life) may have arisen from invasion by micro-organisms in any one of three periods. First, when *in utero* (congenital); secondly, during labour and passage through the birth canal; thirdly, after birth. Some organisms only infect the baby during one of these periods: examples are rubella *in utero* and respiratory syncytial virus (RSV) after birth. Some bacteria may cause infection during more than one of these periods, as is the case with *Streptococcus agalactiae* (group B). A single micro-organism may produce different signs of infection in the infant depending on the period in which it is acquired. For instance, congenital cytomegalovirus (CMV) may result in deafness and microcephaly but postnatally acquired infection in the term infant is generally mild.

The early signs of infection in the neonatal period and early infancy can be subtle and may include only one or two of those given in the following list: pyrexia, low temperature (rectal temperature less than 36.5°C), irritability, floppiness, tachypnoea, apnoea, loss of interest in feeds, disturbance of the normal sleeping pattern. Young infants showing any of these signs may need hospital referral and should not be prescribed antibiotics as this may mask serious infection and complicate diagnosis.

If a doctor is asked to see an infant after the first month with features including fever and nasal discharge, by far the commonest cause is a viral upper-respiratory-tract infection such as coryza. Parents should be asked about the infant's behaviour. Irritability or difficulty in feeding associated with drowsiness may be signs of

more serious infection. The doctor should check carefully for a focus
of infection, paying particular attention to the ears, nose and throat,
and the respiratory rate. The infant should be undressed completely
and examined for evidence of a rash, such as is seen with meningococcal infection. Where the doctor is satisfied that the child
does not require hospital admission, it may be useful to leave
written instructions for the parents. Some practitioners or community services produce printed cards. An example is:

Check the temperature. If over 38° but your child is not getting iller then
keep the room cool; remove most clothing; give some paracetamol (not
aspirin); check your child every 4 hours during the night; **if your child shows
any of the following,** phone . . . immediately:

crying, which you cannot stop by comforting, for more than
two hours;
very rapid breathing (more than 60/min) obtained while the child
is quiet;
a fit or convulsion;
sleepiness or drowsiness that is not a natural sleep;
a rash with what appear to be blood spots in the skin.

Parents may need to be instructed in how to take a temperature
using a conventional thermometer under their child's arm. Many
will not have a mercury thermometer at home. They should be
encouraged to buy one and dissuaded from purchasing a 'strip'
surface thermometer as these frequently underestimate body temperature.

Where the diagnosis is unclear but home management appropriate, the doctor should arrange to check the young febrile infant at a
later time. If a focus of infection is found to account for the fever it
may be appropriate to start an antibiotic; but some arrangements for
follow-up must be made to assess the response to treatment.
Nevertheless, indications for antibiotic treatment in infancy are few
and inappropriate use of these agents—e.g. where there is a possibility, rather than certainty, that otitis media is present, is not
recommended. Such treatment may mask meningitis or prevent
diagnosis of urinary-tract infection with serious consequences. An

exception is where meningococcal disease is suspected. In this case (see p. 96) injection with penicillin may be given prior to transfer to hospital. Unfortunately, the signs of meningitis during infancy are non-specific and can involve changes in the behaviour of the infant, as described above for the neonate. Meningism (a stiff neck) may not occur before 18 months of age; if it does occur early in infancy, it usually implies advanced infection. Also, by 18 months the fontanelle is frequently too small for detection of increased intra-cranial pressure. Because it is difficult to distinguish a febrile convulsion due to meningitis from one associated with a simple virus infection, many paediatricians recommend a lumbar puncture in all infants with a convulsion.

Infants with untreated bacterial infection—meningitis, urinary-tract infection or pneumonia—may deteriorate rapidly and should be referred to a paediatrician where these conditions are suspected. Where the doctor is concerned that the family will be unable to respond to a deterioration should it occur, admission may be justified. If the infant is not admitted to hospital, careful reassessment must be performed in a few hours as circumstances allow. Failure to follow up and check on the often vague non-specific 'warning signals' of infection in infancy is an important error of omission.

The child with respiratory infection

Epidemiology

Infection predominates in any general practice and by far the commonest diagnoses made during childhood are respiratory infections, the common cold, febrile sore throat, and otitis media. Studies of hospital admission rates and patient bed days also show the prominence of respiratory infections and asthma, especially during winter and early spring. Many infections are minor and self-limiting; however, some may represent the early stages of more serious conditions and an important task is to identify these occasional children out of the many who are seen with respiratory symptoms.

Various parts of the respiratory tract may become infected by an enormous range of organisms: viruses, bacteria, chlamydia, mycoplasma species, and fungi. Some infections are responsive to antibiotic therapy which occasionally may be life-saving, but most are caused by viruses and are not susceptible to anti-microbials. Thus, it is important to be as precise as possible in diagnosis to ensure early and effective treatment with antibiotics, while avoiding indiscriminate prescribing. The main sites of respiratory infection with the most important etiological agents to be identified are shown in Table 1.

Nasal passages: the common cold (coryza)

Most children have several colds each year, especially during the winter months, and some never seem to be free from nasal catarrh and a barking cough. When associated allergies and asthma are present their differentiation from an infection may be difficult. During acute episodes of coryza a profuse watery, later purulent nasal discharge is associated with nasal obstruction and mild constitutional symptoms. A blocked nose is particularly trouble-

Table 1 Causes and usual treatment of the main respiratory-tract infections

	Principal agents to be considered	Treatment of bacterial causes
Common cold	rhinoviruses and adenoviruses	
Influenza	influenza viruses	
Pharyngitis/ tonsillitis	*Streptococcus pyogenes* group A (β haemolytic streptococcus) EBV, adenoviruses	penicillin clavulanic acid
Otitis media	*Haemophilus influenzae* type b *S. pneumoniae* (pneumococcus) adenoviruses	amoxycillin amoxycillin
Epiglottitis	*H. influenzae* type b	intubation chloramphenicol amoxycillin
Severe croup	para-influenzae viruses	symptomatic ± intubation
Acute bronchiolitis	respiratory syncytial virus (RSV)	hydration tube-feeding physiotherapy
Pneumonias	viruses bacteria *Chlamydia trachomatis* *Mycoplasma pneumoniae* *Mycobacterium tuberculosis*	initially, penicillin or ampicillin/flucloxacillin ± aminoglycoside or a cephalosporin, e.g. cefotaxime; modified later if specific aetiology identified

some for infants under six months and complicates breathing and feeding. This may be relieved before feeds by gentle nasal cleansing. Short-term relief can also be obtained by nasal decongestants (Otrivine) instilled just before feeding. Paracetamol will relieve constitutional symptoms and reduce irritability. As these infections are caused by rhinoviruses, antibiotics are not indicated and their early use may mask the development of more serious infection and so delay diagnosis.

Pharyngitis and tonsillitis

A febrile illness with a painful, red and inflamed throat and associated lymphadenopathy is common in childhood especially in the early school years. Many of these infections are viral in origin but the main point of diagnostic importance is to identify the presence of group A beta haemolytic streptococci which may initiate the immune complex diseases: glomerulonephritis and rheumatic fever. Bacterial infection is suggested by a fever and an exudate but viruses such as the Epstein–Barr virus (EBV), the cause of glandular fever, may give an identical appearance, and streptococcal infection does not always cause an exudate. Streptococcal infection needs to be treated with an antibiotic, but this selective policy is only feasible where facilities are available for culture from throat swabs. The antibiotic of choice is oral penicillin V, preferably for 10 days and in severe infections the initial dose, or doses, should be given parenterally as benzyl penicillin.

For all forms of tonsillitis or pharyngitis (viral or bacterial) symptomatic treatment with soothing drinks or gargles and an analgesic such as paracetamol are indicated. An exudative tonsillitis or pharyngitis may be caused by EBV. This diagnosis is more likely where there are characteristic punctate haemorrhages on the soft palate in the mouth.

Otitis media

Ears are a frequent site of acute infection in childhood and a careful ear inspection should be part of every examination. This is particularly true for small infants where localizing symptoms and signs may be absent. Fever, vomiting, irritability, or inconsolable crying are the main clinical features. Older children may complain of painful ears, deafness, headache, or dizziness. Fever can be very high and may precipitate a convulsion. Ear examination can show evidence of an acutely inflamed middle ear with prominent vessels on the tympanic membrane (ear-drum), loss of the light reflex from the membrane, and perhaps some distortion or bulging of the drum. A number of organisms cause otitis media, the commonest being: *Haemophilus influenzae* type b, streptococci, pneumococci, and viruses. A broad-spectrum antibiotic, such as amoxycillin, is indicated for infants and children under three years because of the frequency of *H. influenzae* infection, while penicillin remains the drug of choice for older children. Pain and discomfort should be relieved with paracetamol and decongestants. If clinical exudative otitis media ('glue ear') with associated hearing loss persists, a referral to an ear, nose, and throat surgeon or an audiologist is necessary.

Upper-airway obstruction, croup, and epiglottitis

Mild croup of infancy with noisy breathing during the night and improving by day is relatively common. Apart from a cough and perhaps nasal discharge there is usually only a mild constitutional upset. The child's colour remains normal, there is usually only mild respiratory difficulty when the child is upset, and stridor may be absent at rest. These children can usually be treated at home. However, it is the responsibility of the primary-care physician to recognize that children with mild stridor can deteriorate quickly, and those with severe respiratory obstruction caused by laryngo-tracheitis and epiglottitis must be transferred to hospital without delay. Indications for hospital admission include stridor at rest, particularly if the preceding history (usually of sore throat and fever) is short and deterioration has been rapid. There may be other signs of marked respiratory distress such as refusal to eat or drink, with drooling of saliva. In severe obstruction the child appears apprehensive and sits upright, leaning forward in a desperate attempt to aid breathing which is becoming increasingly laboured. With this clinical picture, relief of the obstruction is urgently required.

Obstruction of the airway may be caused by viral inflammatory oedema of the sub-glottic airway (laryngotracheobronchitis) or by inflammation of the epiglottis, usually from infection with *H. influenzae* type b. The history and clinical findings may help to differentiate the two. The child with epiglottitis will have a fever, will appear pale, and will frequently drool. The throat of any child with severe obstruction must not be examined anywhere except in the operating theatre or intensive care, nor should he be disturbed by blood tests or X-rays. It is more important to focus attention on protecting the airway from total obstruction which may be fatal and can occur without warning in a child exhausted by the increased effort of maintaining ventilation. Many hospitals have developed policies for responding to this emergency. Treatment of severe obstruction is by urgent intubation performed by an experienced anaesthetist, with an ENT surgeon present where this is possible because, rarely, a tracheostomy will be required. Blood culture and pharyngeal swabs should be taken after intubation and a parenteral antibiotic effective against *H. influenzae* type b (chloramphenicol or ampicillin) should be given.

If the child's condition is good on admission to hospital and it is agreed that intubation is not required immediately, the child must be nursed where vital signs can be monitored. Frequent (at least half-hourly) observations of colour, heart rate, and respiratory rate, with less frequent measurements of blood gases and pH, will indicate improvement or deterioration within a few hours.

Acute bronchiolitis (see also respiratory syncytial virus p. 109)

This potentially serious infection is common in infants under one year and occurs in epidemics in late winter and early spring. The respiratory syncytial virus (RSV) is responsible for most infections, although other viruses may cause outbreaks. It is a particularly dangerous infection for preterm infants with residual chronic lung disease, and for babies with congenital heart disease and heart failure. Serious outbreaks have been reported from newborn special-care nurseries.

The infection begins like any common cold but a cough, rapid breathing, and wheezing soon develop to the extent that feeding becomes difficult. The characteristic expiratory wheezing results from an inflammatory process causing obstruction of the small airways (bronchioles).

Milder cases show spontaneous improvement after 2–3 days without serious interference with respiration or feeding but in some infants there is progressive breathlessness and cyanosis, continuing hyperinflation of the lungs, widespread moist crepitations, and increasing respiratory acidaemia. Hospitalization is indicated in most such cases, as the baby's condition may deteriorate rapidly and respiratory failure will require assisted ventilation.

RSV can be identified quickly by immunofluorescence of the naso-pharyngeal secretions. This may be helpful in making a decision as to whether antibiotics are required but these may be indicated for a critically ill infant even where RSV has been identified.

General measures in management include tube feeding or even temporary cessation of oral feeding if the infant is critically ill. It is important to maintain adequate hydration if necessary by intra-venous infusion.

Pneumonia in childhood

Although in bacterial pneumonia the causative agent can usually be isolated from the nose or throat, infection is normally confined to the lung. A lobar pneumonia in the child is, for practical purposes, diagnostic of *Streptococcus pneumoniae* (pneumococcus) infection (see p. 103), although it may be seen rarely with *Staphylococcus aureus* infection (see p. 121). Pneumonia associated with effusion is generally caused by *S. pneumoniae*, and less commonly *S. aureus*. Viral infections of the upper respiratory tract may be associated with pneumonia.

Chlamydia trachomatis pneumonia (see p. 46) should be considered in the young infant, as should be bacterial pathogens such as *Streptococcus pneumoniae* (pneumococcus), *Staphylococcus aureus*, and *Haemophilus influenzae* (see p. 70). The bacterial agents are seen throughout childhood, although *Mycoplasma pneumoniae* is unusual under the age of five, while being responsible for up to 20 per cent of cases in school-age children. Tuberculosis must be considered in the differential diagnosis of lower-respiratory-tract infection, especially in recently arrived immigrant children. Immunocompromized children are particularly susceptible to infection with *Pneumocystis carinii* and fungi such as *Candida* sp.

In young children the presentation of pneumonia can be subtle. There may be no obvious respiratory distress, although there will usually be tachypnoea and tachycardia. Added sounds and other clinical findings useful in adults may be absent on auscultation. The diagnosis should be suspected in infants with fever, grunting, nasal flaring, and tachypnoea, perhaps in association with drowsiness and irritability when disturbed (features suggestive of hypoxaemia). In older children, especially if the pneumonia involves the lower segments of the lung, abdominal pain may be the presenting feature. Right upper-lobe pneumonia can cause neck stiffness without any chest signs and hence masquerade as meningitis.

In almost all circumstances hospitalization is indicated, particularly in infants, as respiratory failure needs to be anticipated and treated. In management, general measures include the provision of humidified oxygen sufficient to maintain adequate oxygenation. If feeding has ceased or is considered dangerous (because of possible aspiration), an intravenous infusion will be necessary to maintain hydration and also provide a convenient access for drugs. Physiotherapy is important where there is extensive consolidation.

Although in many cases a viral aetiology is likely, an antibiotic is usually prescribed, as delay in starting effective therapy can have serious consequences. The pattern of onset, clinical findings, chest X-ray appearances, the leucocyte count and its differential may be helpful in determining the most appropriate antibiotic. When a bacterial pneumonia is suspected, a set of blood cultures should be taken and antibiotic treatment reviewed when the results are available. In early childhood the most likely bacterial pathogens are *S. pneumoniae* and *H. influenzae* type b, but staphylococcal pneumonia should be considered when the initial chest X-ray shows extensive consolidation.

The child with a rash

This section outlines the diagnostic process applied to a child presenting with a rash of rapid onset. Rare causes are not included; the conditions described will, however, cover almost all cases encountered in community practice and in the majority of hospital referrals. Some common rashes of non-infectious aetiology are also included. The management of most of the infectious causes is covered under the named illnesses; however, a few infections are too minor to deserve separate consideration and are covered within this section.

Many rashes look similar and the diagnosis is not based on appearance alone. A history and general examination are essential and a schema for this is as follows.

History

prior infectious diseases and/or rashes,
recent contact with infectious disease,
prior and recent immunizations,
foreign travel,
present and recent medication,
prodromal illness (symptoms appearing prior to rash) especially fever,
similar illnesses occurring in the locality,
itch.

General examination

general state,
temperature,
lymphadenopathy,
splenomegaly,
conjunctivae,

respiratory signs,
signs on the mouth (e.g. Koplik's spots in measles) and ears.

Features of the rash

What form does it take?

Vesicular (fluid-filled sacs);
Maculopapular (a mixture of macules—flat lesions, and papules
   —raised; as in measles);
Punctiform (pinpoint-like) as in rubella;
Haemorraghic (petechiae, which are small, or the larger ecchymoses)

Over which part of the body was the rash first seen? What is its
present distribution? Is there evidence of scratching?

Rashes in well babies

In community practice healthy young children, and particularly
babies, frequently present with trivial punctiform, maculopapular
and even vesicular rashes. During the neonatal period many infants
develop an erythematous and sometimes vesicular rash (erythema
toxicum, neonatal urticaria). These lesions are sometimes confused
with the uncommon but potentially serious staphylococcal sepsis
(pemphigus). Where there is doubt the contents of a vesicle should
be smeared on a microscope slide and a Gram stain performed.
Eosinophils will be seen in cases of neonatal urticaria and Gram-
positive cocci in pemphigus. When micro-organisms are seen, a
culture should be collected and the infant started on antibiotics.
Otherwise, it is important to check that the baby is apyrexial,
feeding well, and that there are no signs of local infection. In these
cases, simple reassurance is indicated.

Causes of vesicular rashes

chickenpox;
dermatitis herpetiformis;
hand, foot, and mouth disease;

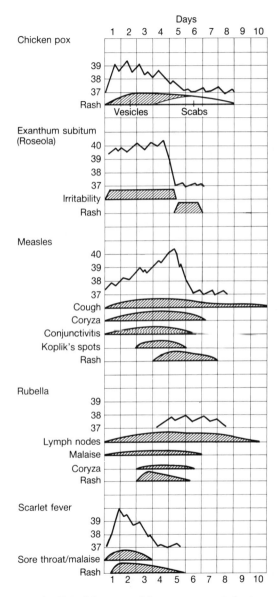

Fig. 2 Diagnostic clinical features of five commoner infections causing a rash.

herpes simplex and eczema herpeticum;
herpes zoster;
impetigo;
insect bites;
molluscum contagiosum.

(Note: drug eruptions and allergic reactions can, but rarely do, cause vesicular rashes.)

The important diagnostic features of conditions associated with rashes are tabulated in Table 2 and described below where the condition is not covered in the Diseases section.

Dermatitis herpetiformis

There is no prodromal illness or general malaise but symmetrical erythematous itchy vesicles appear gradually over the trunk, eventually resolving leaving dark pigmentation (or depigmentation on Asian or black skin).

Eczema herpeticum

The child has a history of eczema, sometimes of cold sores, is acutely unwell with fever and vesicular lesions in the eczematous areas.

Insect bites

Generally painful or itchy with an erythematous base but rarely with systemic disturbance.

Causes of maculopapular and punctiform rashes

enteroviral infections,
erythema infectiosum (fifth disease),
exanthem subitum (roseola infantum),
infectious mononucleosis,
measles,
meningococcal disease,
Kawasaki disease (mucocutaneous lymph node syndrome)

Table 2 Diagnostic features of common rashes

	Prodrome	Fever	General malaise	Distribution of rash	Itchy	Special features
Vesicular rashes						
Chickenpox	Non or short coryzal	Mild	Mild	Mostly trunk	Yes	Contact with other sufferers is common; crops
Dermatitis herpetiformis	Nil	Nil	Nil	Trunk	Yes	Sporadic cases eventually leave depigmentation
Eczema herpeticum	Nil	Moderate	Moderate	In areas of eczema	Yes	May be seriously ill
Hand, foot, and mouth	Nil	Minimal	Minimal	Palm, soles, and inside mouth	No	Often in minor epidemics
H. simplex (gingivo-stomatitis)	Nil	Mild	Moderate	Mouth and lips	Yes	Frequent history of contact with cold sores
Impetigo	Nil	Nil	Nil	Face and hands	Yes	Vesicles often replaced by yellow eruptions
Insect bites	Nil	Nil	Rare	Variable	Yes	Usually isolated lesions
Molluscum contagiosum	Nil	Nil	Nil	Variable	No	Characteristic pearly vesicles with central dimple

Table 2 Diagnostic features of common rashes (*contd*)

	Prodrome	Fever	General malaise	Distribution of rash	Itchy	Special features
Maculopapular and punctiform rashes						
Enteroviral infections	Short	Very mild	Mild	General	No	
Erythema infectiosum (Fifth disease, slapped cheeks syndrome)	Uncommon mild fever and respiratory symptoms	Mild if any	Minimal	Face 'slapped cheeks' and limbs	No	—
Exanthem subitum (roseola infantum, sixth disease)	High fever and irritability	High	Substantial	Trunk then face	No	The child improves dramatically when rash appears on 4th or 5th day
Glandular fever	Malaise, mild fever, and sore throat	Moderate	Common	General	No	Exudate in throat especially marked
Measles	Rising fever, cough, conjunctivitis	High	Substantial	Around ears then face, then trunk; confluent	No	Koplik's spots in mouth before rash on 4th day of illness

Disease	Prodrome		Toxicity	Distribution		Features
Meningococcal disease	None or short with coryza or fever	Variable	Profound	Variable	No	Maculopapular rash may precede petechial rash
Kawasaki disease (Mucocutaneous lymph node syndrome)	Mild fever, malaise, sore throat	Mild	Mild to moderate	General	No	Palms and soles, lips and conjunctivae affected
Pityriasis rosea	Nil	Nil	Nil	Trunk	Initially	Usually older children; herald patch at onset
Rubella	Short, mild fever and malaise	Mild	Mild or nil	Face then trunk and limbs	No	Posterior occipital lymphadenopathy
Scarlet fever	Fever and sore throat	Yes	Moderate	Face then rapidly generalized	No	Rash blanches on pressure; strawberry tongue and peri-oral pallor

pityriasis rosea,
rubella,
scarlet fever.

(Note also: drug eruptions, malaria, sunburn, and contact allergies can cause maculopapular or punctiform rashes.)

The important diagnostic features are tabulated in Table 2 and described below where the condition is not covered in the Diseases section. See also Fig. 2, p. 15.

Enteroviral infections

A number of these viruses (coxsackie, echoviruses) produce a very mild fever and malaise which may precede, but more often coincide with the rash which is discrete (i.e. the macules do not run into one another), non-itchy and general in distribution.

Exanthem subitum (roseola infantum)

A disease showing a continuous high fever (up to 40°C) and irritability, which both subside with the appearance of a discrete maculopapular rash at 4–5 days. This is initially on the trunk and then spreads to the face and limbs. (See also p. 000 and Fig. 2.)

Pityriasis rosea

This occurs in older (school-age) children. Initially a patch appears on the trunk looking like ringworm (the herald patch). Later there are more generalized red papules which merge to form an oval plaque which is initially itchy. This condition is not infectious to others.

Causes of haemorrhagic rashes

The rapid onset of a haemorrhagic rash suggests either meningococcal infection or a clotting disorder (e.g. idiopathic thrombocytopaenic purpura (ITP) or leukaemia). Urgent referral is necessary.

Other rashes

Scabies

This produces an itchy rash sometimes with papules and vesicles, most common around fingers, wrists and elbows. Linear burrows may be seen but are frequently hidden by the frantic scratching. Other family members are often affected. (See also p. 000.)

Itchy rashes

Itchiness and scratching are characteristic of the following:

chickenpox;
eczema;
hand, foot, and mouth disease;
herpes simplex;
impetigo;
insect bites.

The child with a fever

This section deals with cases in which the major, perhaps the only, presenting feature is a fever. Acute pyrexia will be considered first followed by persistent fever (pyrexia of unknown origin—PUO).

Acute fever

The commonest causes are (in approximately diminishing frequency): acute viral illness (various types); otitis media; tonsillitis; pneumonia; gastroenteritis; urinary-tract infection; bacteraemia; infectious hepatitis; meningitis; malaria; non-infectious conditions, e.g. connective tissue disorders.

A careful history has to be taken with emphasis on recent general health, other symptoms, contact with infections, travel abroad, and, in particular, present medication. A thorough examination must be performed to identify the more common infections. This will include ears, conjunctivae, throat, neck (for stiffness), chest, lymph nodes, and abdomen. (Palpation of a spleen may reveal that the 'tonsillitis' is in reality part of glandular fever.) The child must be undressed completely so that any rash may be observed.

If the child is only moderately unwell with signs of a viral infection (lymphadenopathy, injected conjunctivae, inflamed fauces, and rash) home care with symptomatic treatment can be given. Red eyes and ear-drums may arise from persistent crying rather than infection. Otitis media may be hard to diagnose because of difficulty in viewing the tympanic membranes. Where this is suspected but not confirmed the child should be re-examined later.

When no diagnosis can be made, but the child is obviously unwell, the more serious causes must be excluded by further examination (bones, joints, and soft tissues). A specific diagnosis may be particularly difficult to make in very young children (see p. 3) or if an antibiotic has already been given which could mask a serious infection. In these circumstances, referral to hospital is recommended. Where there is no obvious focus of infection in infancy or childhood, urinary-tract infection should be considered and a urine specimen collected (see p. 25). It may be necessary to review the child in a few hours.

If a decision is made to treat a baby or child at home, the family need instructions in how to manage a fever, the signs of deterioration, and what actions to take. These are best written down; some practitioners supply standard cards (as described on p. 4).

Persistent fever—PUO (pyrexia of unknown origin)

Technically this is defined as a temperature (over 38.5°C) lasting for more than 14 days without a diagnosis. However, any child with a fever for more than five days with no obvious cause requires referral to hospital. Infectious aetiologies remain the commonest causes of PUO; but fever may be a component of other illnesses.

Again, history and examination should be scrupulous. Investigations will depend on the clinical findings but must include urine microscopy and culture, full blood count and film, blood cultures, and, if the child has been to a malarious country, even if prophylaxis was given, a thick blood film.

Causes of persistent fever

Infective causes

Abscesses (dental, osteomyelitis, peritonsillar, appendix); bacteraemia; septic arthritis; endocarditis; infective hepatitis; glandular fever (infectious mononucleosis); Kawasaki disease (mucocutaneous lymph node syndrome); sinusitis; tuberculosis; typhoid fever; urinary-tract infection; listeriosis; brucellosis; malaria (foreign travel); relapsing fever (foreign travel).

Non-infective causes

Uncommon causes

Malignancy: leukaemia, lymphomas; gastrointestinal: ulcerative colitis, Crohn's disease; connective tissue disorders: systemic juvenile rheumatoid arthritis (Still's disease); antibiotic induced.

Rare causes

Malignancy: sarcoma, histiocytosis; connective tissue disorders: systemic lupus erythematosus (SLE), Behcet's syndrome, ectodermal dysplasia; factitious: Munchausen by proxy syndrome; neurodegenerative disorders.

The child with urinary-tract infection

The diagnosis of urinary-tract infection (UTI) should be considered in any infant or child with fever, especially with rigors or vomiting. Dysuria, while a common symptom in the older child, cannot be declared under the age of two, and frequency is unlikely to be noted in the normally incontinent infant. Infection should be considered in the presence of nocturnal enuresis or when an established toiletting pattern breaks down.

Diagnosis is important, particularly under the age of five, because untreated infection in the presence of ureteric reflux may lead to renal scarring which, when severe, may progress to end-stage renal failure in later years. Early treatment should reduce the likelihood of renal damage.

Because it is so important to exclude UTI in a child with fever, antibiotics should not be given unless there is an obvious cause of infection (e.g. tonsillitis, pneumonia). The diagnosis of a suspected first UTI must be confirmed by microscopy and culture (testing for protein alone is unacceptable). If a urine specimen is not collected and sent to the laboratory for culture an important congenital renal abnormality may be missed. Furthermore, a paediatrician may subsequently be uncertain as to whether or not the child has had a urinary-tract infection and may feel obliged to arrange what can be unnecessary investigation. However, it is normal practice for paediatricians to arrange radiological investigations in all children under the age of one year following a single urinary-tract infection, and to investigate after either one or two infections in children up to the age of six.

During infancy the satisfactory collection of urine is a fine art. Clean catch specimens are probably best but require time, patience, and an appropriate receptacle (sterile jar) to hand. Urine specimens are frequently collected in adhesive sterile, disposable bags applied

to the skin around the perineum. The perineum should be washed
with water before the bag is applied. This is best done in a warm
room with the bag exposed and the infant held upright so that as
soon as urine is passed the bag can be removed and urine drained
from a freshly cut hole into a sterile container. False negatives are
uncommon using this technique but a high proportion of false
positives will occur if the bag is left on too long, allowing
contamination with bacteria from the perineal skin. In the toilet-
trained child, specimens can be collected successfully from a clean
potty, and in older children an MSU (see p. 159) can be taken.

Specimens should be sent to the laboratory immediately after
collection. Failing this, they can be kept in a refrigerator (at 4°C) and
sent the next day. When only a culture result is required a dipslide
can be used: a plastic paddle coated with agar is dipped into the
urine and then sent to the laboratory.

Urinary-tract infection can be diagnosed when a single bacterial
strain is cultured with a count of 10^5 organisms/ml, or more. Most
infections are associated with pyuria, that is more than 50 leucocytes
(white blood cells) on microscopy. When this is the first occasion
that infection is suspected in a young child, and the specimen has
been collected into a bag, another sample should be obtained to
confirm infection before antibiotics are given. This should be done
by suprapubic aspiration in hospital, or clean catch. The specimen
should be collected quickly, particularly in infancy when urinary
infection can progress to septicaemia over a short period. Indeed, in
a sick infant with suspected urinary-tract infection there is no place
for a bag urine collection and a suprapubic aspiration of urine
should be performed. In an older child with pyelonephritis (dysuria,
fever, loin tenderness) there is less need for a second sample. A
second sample should also be taken if there is a positive culture, but
normal urine microscopy.

Most urinary-tract infections in children are caused by Gram-
negative bowel commensals, especially *Escherichia coli*. When
antibiotics need to be given before the culture results are available,
trimethoprin or co-trimoxazole (sulphamethoxazole and trimethoprin) are the drugs of choice. Other antibiotics may be required once
the results of sensitivity testing are available (amoxycillin, cephra-

dine and nitrofurantoin). Antibiotic treatment should continue for five days.

Prophylactic antibiotic treatment may be given to some infants and young children thought to be at risk of further infection, particularly where there are known to be congenital renal abnormalities or where ureteric reflux has been demonstrated by investigation. A urine culture should be performed 3–5 days after treatment has been discontinued, or during prophylactic treatment. Care should be taken with the interpretation of urine results in children on antibiotics; pyuria alone may be the only indication that infection is still present. Children with a first infection, particularly under the age of five, should be referred to a paediatrician who will then decide on further investigations; referral should be urgent in children under the age of one year, who will need a suprapubic aspiration or clean-catch urine collection as soon as a urinary infection is thought to be present.

The parents of children with UTIs should be advised to encourage plentiful fluids during episodes of infection. Careful attention should be paid to toilet hygiene, and bubble baths, which may promote irritation and lead to further infection, should be discouraged, particularly for girls.

The child with vomiting and diarrhoea

Vomiting

The commonest cause of vomiting is gastrointestinal infection and is often associated with diarrhoea. Vomiting may be a symptom of other childhood conditions which may need urgent investigation and treatment, such as meningitis and urinary-tract infection.

Causes other than gastroenteritis to be considered are listed below.

Vomiting of central origin

Meningitis, encephalitis, intracranial-space-occupying lesion, migraine, Reye's syndrome.

Vomiting from gastrointestinal disease

(1) In the newborn: intestinal obstruction from small-bowel atresia, meconium ileus, Hirschsprung's disease, malrotation, volvulus;
(2) in infancy: pyloric stenosis, intussusception, appendicitis, oesophageal hiatus hernia;
(3) in childhood: appendicitis, malrotation, oesophageal stricture.

Metabolic causes

Congenital adrenal hyperplasia, Addison's disease, diabetic keto-acidosis, uraemia in renal failure.

Other causes

Drugs and toxins, periodic syndrome, pregnancy in adolescent girls, as part of systemic infections, tonsillitis, otitis media, urinary-tract infection, measles, hepatitis.

The causes listed above should be considered and eliminated by careful history and examination before a diagnosis of gastroenteritis is made. For instance a vomiting child with fever and neck stiffness is likely to have meningitis, fever with rigors urinary tract infection, and where the vomiting is bile stained intestinal obstruction is likely.

When the child appears unwell and there is no clear cause referral to hospital may be indicated. This is the case for persistent vomiting, particularly in infancy, which may lead quickly to electrolyte imbalance. **There is no place for anti-emetic drugs in the vomiting child.**

Diarrhoea

In early infancy babies (especially if breast fed) may have frequent soft even watery stools. Older children can have 'toddler diarrhoea' (persistent loose stools containing undigested food in a well child growing normally).

Diarrhoea is rarely due to disease beyond the gastro-intestinal tract. Although most causes of acute change in bowel habit are due to local infections the causes listed below need to be considered particularly where the diarrhoea is prolonged. A useful sign is that with the exception of malabsorptive conditions (eg cystic fibrosis) foul-smelling stools generally indicate infection.

Conditions where diarrhoea can be a presenting feature

(1) During infancy: drugs (especially antibiotics), lactose or cows' milk protein intolerance, urinary-tract infection, coeliac disease, cystic fibrosis, appendicitis;

(2) during childhood: drugs, laxatives; appendicitis; ulcerative colitis; Crohn's disease; haemolytic uraemic syndrome; mucocutaneous lymph node syndrome (Kawasaki disease).

For both vomiting and/or diarrhoea, once a diagnosis of gastroenteritis has been made, further management should proceed as described on p. 58–61.

The child with sexually transmitted disease

Microbiological tests and their use in providing possible evidence of sexual abuse

Evidence for sexually transmitted diseases may be sought in children suffering from anal, penile, and vaginal warts, vaginal or urethral discharges or when there is a history of contact with an individual with a known or possible genital infection. The recommended investigations are summarized in Table 3. Where genital warts are seen, it is recommended that they are removed (under general anaesthesia in the young child) and sent for typing. Rapid diagnostic tests for *Chlamydia trachomatis*, such as the enzyme-linked immunosorbent assay (ELISA) and immunofluorescence, may be unreliable and the diagnosis should be confirmed by cell culture. Results of *Neisseria gonorrhoeae* culture may need to be confirmed by a reference laboratory.

Gonorrhoea, perianal warts, and *Chlamydia* infections outside the immediate newborn period are strongly suggestive of sexual contact. If child sexual abuse is suspected, then it is important that the specimens are handled to meet the requirements for collecting forensic evidence, that is, the person who takes the specimen and all subsequent people who handle it should sign the label to ensure continuity of evidence. If child sexual abuse is suspected, it would be appropriate for the child to be assessed by a doctor with relevant experience. It is currently recommended that a full examination in a paediatric setting is performed by a paediatrician and an experienced police surgeon.

For a more detailed discussion of *N. gonorrhoeae* infection see p. 66–7; for *C. trachomatis* see p. 46–7; and herpes simplex virus p. 80–2.

Table 3 Investigations to be performed for diagnosis of sexually transmitted agents in childhood; detection of one or more of these agents from the genital tract in infancy or childhood indicates probable sexual abuse

Organism/lesion	Site of specimen	Transport to laboratory on	Recommended isolation/confirmation	Comments
Neisseria gonorrhoeae	vagina penile urethra anus fauces	charcoal swab	culture on agar	
Chlamydia trachomatis	vagina penile urethra anus (remove pus before specimen collected)	swab in Chlamydia transport medium and smear on microscope slide	cell culture immunofluorescence	Always confirm with culture if rapid diagnostic test is positive
Trichomonas vaginalis	vagina	charcoal swab or trichomonas culture medium	microscopy culture	
Herpes simplex virus (HSV)/genital herpes	vagina penile urethra anus	swab in viral transport medium	tissue culture electron microscopy	Reactivation of lesions occurs
Human papilloma virus (HPV), condyloma acuminata (wart)	anus vagina penis	rapid transit and freeze at −70°C (biopsy specimen)	histology electron microscopy	DNA analysis may be available for identification of genital HPV strains

Congenital infections

Management of important infections during pregnancy and the neonatal period

Table 4

Organism/ disease	Management in pregnancy	Management of new-born
Chlamydia trachomatis	Treat parents with erythromycin	Tetracycline to eyes, oral erythromycin
Cytomegalovirus (CMV)	Rarely diagnosed; symptoms milds	Symptomatic
Enterovirus	No action if in early pregnancy	Isolate newborn from other infants where intra-partum infection
Hepatitis B	—	Hepatitis B immune globulin and vaccine where mother HBeAg positive and anti-HBe negative (see p. 193); increasing tendency to immunize all HBsAg mothers; barrier nurse (see Glossary) where mother e antigen positive
Herpes simplex virus (HSV) (genital)	Greatest risk in 1° infection; Caesarean section where lesions present	Acyclovir in definite or suspected infection; isolate
Human immuno-deficiency virus (HIV) AIDS/ARC	Consider termination of pregnancy because of high risk of congenital infection	Isolation unnecessary; extreme care with blood (see p. 41)

Organism/ disease	Management in pregnancy	Management of new-born
Listeria mono-cytogenes Listeriosis	Ampicillin 4–6 g/day in acute infection	Penicillin or ampicillin in high doses
Measles	No action required	— (Extremely rare)
Mumps	No action required	— (Extremely rare)
Mycobacterium tuberculosis/ Tuberculosis (TB)	Positive tuberculin test and positive CXR needs treatment	Isolate infant from mother with active TB and give isoniazid (INAH) and INAH-resistant BCG; give INAH and rifampicin to infant with TB
Neisseria gonorrhoea/ gonorrhoea	Ampicillin or benzyl penicillin im or iv	Single dose of benzyl penicillin where untreated maternal infection and asymptomatic infant; treat neonatal infection with benzyl penicillin iv for seven days
Rubella*	Counsel for possible termination following infection before 18 weeks' gestation	Symptomatic; early hearing tests
Streptococcus agalactiae Group B	Ampicillin 2 g every 4 h where amnionitis and where colonized	Benzyl penicillin intravenously
Toxoplasma gondii/ toxoplasmosis	Rarely diagnosed (see p. 136–8) Spiramycin	Courses of pyrimethamine, sulphadiazine, folinic acid, and spiramycin (see p. 138)
Treponema pallidum/ Syphilis	Treat with benzyl penicillin, (a) clinical disease +/− pos VDRL (venereal disease research laboratory)	

Organism/ disease	Management in pregnancy	Management of new-born
	(b) and pos VDRL with pos FTA-ABS (fluorescent treponemal antibody)	
Varicella/ chickenpox	Zoster immuno-globulin (ZIG) for infection in early pregnancy, or seronegative mother exposed to infection; termination of pregnancy not indicated	ZIG where maternal infection 5 days before to 7 days after delivery; give acyclovir alone for neonatal infection; observe for 10 days after onset of rash in mother; infants at highest risk with rash 5–10 days after birth

Breast feeding should be encouraged for infants with congenital infection. Although HIV has been isolated from breast milk there is no evidence that infection has been transmitted to the newborn, except where infection has been acquired postnatally. In the UK, where infants cows' milk formulae are available, artificial feeding may be preferred.

*To diagnose acute maternal rubella infection provide paired sera to demonstrate rise in rubella antibody, the first taken within 2–3 days of onset of the rash and the second from 8–9 days after the onset; alternatively provide a single sample from seven days to six weeks after the onset for estimation of rubella-specific IgM. Provide the laboratory with a full clinical history. All suspected cases of congenital rubella syndrome must be notified to the National Congenital Rubella Surveillance Scheme (see p. 118).

Diseases

AIDS (Acquired immunodeficiency syndrome)/HIV infection

Organism

The human immunodeficiency virus (HIV).

Epidemiology

AIDS is not a notifiable disease and figures are based on laboratory reports of HIV-positive results and voluntary clinical case reporting to the British Paediatric Surveillance Unit (BPSU), the Communicable Disease Surveillance Centre (CDSC), or the Communicable Disease Unit (Scotland). Paediatricians and other doctors managing HIV positive children and paediatric AIDS cases should ensure that they are reported to the relevant body.

By the end of December 1987 there had been 253 laboratory reports in the UK of children (under age 15) having blood positive for antibody to HIV (see Table 4). In addition, 21 cases of childhood AIDS had been reported to the BPSU to August 1987, as meeting the case definition on 2 April 1988 (Table 6).

The two main groups of children infected in the UK were cases where transmission was from mother to child (vertical transmission) and others infected by transfusion of blood products or blood itself. In addition, there are a small number of paediatric AIDS cases where transmission occurred outside the UK and others where information is insufficient to determine the route of infection.

The most important source of infection in a child is from its mother. Women at highest risk of HIV infection are:

- drug abusers who have injected themselves since 1977;
- sexual partners of such drug abusers;

Table 5 Paediatric HIV-antibody positive reports to December 1987

Transmission/exposure category	Residents in UK			
	0–4 yrs	5–9 yrs	10–14 yrs	Total
Parent HIV infected or in risk group	82	1	—	83
Blood-component recipients:				
abroad	1	—	—	1
UK	—	—	1	1
undetermined	—	2	1	3
haemophiliac	10	62	87	159
Others/undetermined	3	—	3	6
Total	96	65	92	253

- sexual partners of bisexual men;
- women who had a transfusion or sex with men living in Africa south of the countries bordering on the Mediterranean in countries where AIDS is endemic;
- prostitutes;
- sexual partners of haemophiliacs.

The majority of women in the above risk groups will not be infected. Also, women may not realize that they are within the risk groups, and HIV infection occurs in women outside of these groups. The highest risk is amongst women associated with injected drug abuse, amongst whom HIV-infection prevalence varies geographically. There is a particularly high rate, and hence a concentration of infected children, in Lothian (Scotland).

Transmission

Vertical transmission is the commonest source of new cases of HIV infection. Prenatal transmission occurs and transmission at birth through exposure to maternal blood seems likely. The role of breast feeding is under study. Kissing, close proximity, and other casual

Table 6 Paediatric AIDS cases to December 1987

Transmission/exposure category	Residents in UK			Visitors	Total
	0–4 yrs	5–9 yrs	10–14 yrs	0–14 yrs	
Parent HIV infected or in risk group	6	1	—	6	13
Blood-component recipients:					
abroad	1	1	—	2	4
UK	—	—	—	—	—
haemophiliac	—	1	1	—	2
Total	7	3	1	8	19

Figures, supplied by CDSC, include those for Scotland (note: AIDS totals slightly at variance with BPSU).

contacts do **NOT** lead to infection. With the exclusion of high-risk donors, the screening of donated blood for antibody as well as heat treatment of some blood products (Factor VIII), the risk of HIV infection following transfusion is very low. Infection can be transmitted following transfusion of infected blood before sero conversion of the donor has occurred.

Incubation period

(from exposure to antibody production) in adults infected by transfusion is approximately six weeks (median period); much longer periods have been reported in some children.

Infectivity

Apart from through the transfusion and vertical routes, infectivity is very low, considerably less than for hepatitis B. It is important for HIV-positive children to be treated as other children, and it must be appreciated that properly applied normal standards of infection control will prevent spread of the disease in the hospital and community. The Multicentre European Study has found a vertical transmission rate of approximately 25 per cent, with indications that women with symptomatic HIV infection are more likely to have infected babies.

Natural history

There is a spectrum of HIV infection from entirely asymptomatic cases through to AIDS itself. The majority of children infected through transfusion have developed some abnormality, and the median time from transfusion to AIDS is estimated to be two years. The manifestations of HIV infection in children are variable and considerably different from adults. Children who become symptomatic may present with any one or a combination of the following: recurrent bacterial infections, failure to thrive, persistent and recurrent severe oral candida (thrush), persistent or recurrent diarrhoea, generalized lymphadenopathy, enlarged liver and spleen (hepatosplenomegaly), progressive encephalopathy, or loss of developmental milestones.

Diagnosis

Because of the persistence of maternal antibody it is particularly difficult to diagnose HIV infection in children under 15 months. Virus isolation or antigen detection can help but is usually only available in specialist centres. Children found to be HIV positive under 15 months but who are asymptomatic, have no immunological abnormalities, and have not had isolation of virus or antigen detection, are referred to as having 'indeterminate' status. Conventional antibody testing is usually by an ELISA but a positive result must then be confirmed by a second independent test (using either another type of ELISA or a Western blot test). For these and other reasons, diagnosis of both HIV positivity and paediatric AIDS is complicated and specialist advice must be sought.

See p. 257 for immunization of HIV-positive children.

Childhood HIV infection has only been recognized in the past few years and knowledge about it is rapidly accumulating. Hence, policy on management and care are changing and are not appropriate for detailed discussion in a book such as this. Readers are advised to consult the guidelines published by the Royal College of Obstetricians and Gynaecologists and the British Paediatric Association (Further reading, nos 18 and 19, p. 333). Recommendations include the following:

Childbirth

Gloves, gowns, masks, and goggles should be used by staff assisting in childbirth when a woman is known to be HIV positive, or is in a high risk group.

Staff with open wounds or eczema on the hands should cover the affected areas with waterproof plasters or gloves when caring for a high risk mother in childbirth, or her infant.

Paediatricians attending high risk deliveries should wear masks, disposable gowns, surgical gloves, and safety spectacles.

Only mechanical suction should be used. The infant should be washed free of blood and liquor after delivery.

Careful attention should be paid to disinfection of non-disposable apparatus (1 per cent sodium hypochlorite to be used).

The infant receiving intensive care

Extreme care should be used in practical procedures such as venesection and insertion of catheters into blood vessels. Staff should cover open wounds on their hands and when feasible gloves should be worn.

Breast feeding

It is suggested that HIV positive mothers in the UK should bottle feed their infants. However there is no evidence to suggest that breast feeding increases the risk of transmission of infection to the newborn, except in the very rare cases of postnatally acquired infection. This recommendation should not be adopted in developing countries, where women should be encouraged to breast feed.

Immunization

BCG should not be given to an HIV positive infant, or to an infant of an HIV positive mother.

Oral polio vaccine (OPV) can be given to an HIV positive infant. However, if another member of the family is immunocompromised killed polio vaccine (IPV) should be used.

Measles vaccine and the measles, mumps, rubella vaccine (MMR) should be administered to HIV positive infants.

Diphtheria, pertussis and tetanus vaccines are indicated.

Chickenpox (varicella) and Herpes zoster (shingles)

Organism

Herpes virus—varicella/zoster; a DNA virus.

Epidemiology

Chickenpox is highly infectious so that most children become infected and remain immune into adulthood. Infection in childhood is normally benign but may be severe in the immuno-suppressed child, and in the newborn infant when infection develops in the mother close to the time of delivery.

Transmission

is by direct contact, droplet infection or recently soiled materials, e.g. handkerchiefs.

Incubation period

is from 14 to 21 days.

Period of infectivity

is from one day prior to eruption of the rash and then for six days after the rash appears.

Natural history of infection in childhood and pregnancy

Primary infection with the virus results in chickenpox. There may be a short (less than 24 hours) coryzal prodrome followed by fever and an itchy vesicular rash. Crops of vesicles, sparser on the limbs than trunk, appear over 3–5 days.

Complications are unusual but include thrombocytopenia and encephalitis. Aspirin given during this illness is thought to increase the risk of Reye's syndrome. Immunosuppressed children have continued cropping of lesions as well as encephalitis, pancreatitis, hepatitis, and pneumonia. Infection during early pregnancy may result in varicella embryopathy, but this is extremely rare and does not justify termination of pregnancy.

Reactivation of the virus which lies latent in a spinal nerve root may occur in both children and adults, and results in shingles or zoster, a painful rash where vesicles are grouped in a dermatome pattern (a dermatome is an area of skin served by a single spinal nerve).

Diagnosis

The diagnosis should be made on clinical features, but virus in vesicle fluid can be identified by electron microscopy or virus culture.

Management

Symptomatic treatment only is required in childhood **but aspirin should never be used as an antipyretic**. Children with chickenpox should not be admitted to hospital unless absolutely necessary because of the risk to immunosuppressed children. Infants and children with varicella should be barrier nursed.

The immunosuppressed child should be given zoster immune globulin (ZIG) if known to be varicella seronegative and in close contact with a case. (Management will need to be discussed with a paediatrician.) If lesions appear, then oral acyclovir should be used; ZIG is of no value at this stage. Where pregnant women are exposed to varicella–zoster and they are susceptible then ZIG should be given.

Neonatal varicella—natural history and treatment

This is rare and babies are only at risk when the mother develops chickenpox between five days before and seven days after delivery. It presents as a vesicular rash and there is a high mortality from varicella pneumonia. ZIG should be given to the newborn if the mother develops varicella during the risk period. Acyclovir (intravenous or oral) is indicated following development of lesions in the newborn and is sometimes used in the mother and in her baby prophylactically where maternal infection occurs just before delivery.

Chlamydia trachomatis

C. trachomatis ophthalmia neonatorum is notifiable

Organism

Chlamydia trachomatis. Some serotypes cause endemic trachoma and others sexually transmitted infections. This is a bacterial agent with an intra-cellular life cycle.

Epidemiology

This is the commonest cause of sexually transmitted infection in the UK. Infection is acquired during sexual intercourse or parturition. If the mother is infected, up to 50 per cent of infants develop conjunctivitis after delivery and almost half of untreated infants with conjunctivitis will develop pneumonia. *C. trachomatis* ophthalmia is more common than that due to the gonococcus and is notifiable. Identification in the genital tract of children implies sexual abuse.

Natural history

A purulent neonatal conjunctivitis may develop 5–14 days after birth and cannot be distinguished on clinical appearances from gonococcal or other infection. Inadequate treatment may result in recurrence and, rarely, in corneal scarring. Pneumonia may develop 4–6 weeks after birth and is associated with poor feeding, a cough, and tachypnoea. The chest X-ray shows hyper-inflation and generalized patchy shadowing. Pneumonia, although requiring treatment, is often self-limiting, but the outcome may be more serious in the preterm infant with coexistent chronic lung disease (bronchopulmonary dysplasia). Infection in the adolescent may lead to non-specific/non-gonococcal urethritis (NSU, NGU) and, in the female, salpingitis and possible infertility.

Diagnosis

A Gram stain on the exudate should be performed immediately (day or night) in all cases of purulent conjunctivitis, to exclude gonococcal infection. Because *C. trachomatis* is an intra-cellular bacterium the specimen should include cells from the conjunctivae collected by firmly drawing a cotton-wool swab over the everted lower eyelid. Rapid diagnostic tests using monoclonal antibodies have been introduced and allow diagnosis of *C. trachomatis* from a smear on a microscope slide. An enzyme-linked immunosorbent assay is also available (ELISA). All these tests, but particularly the ELISA, may yield false positive results and for this reason the definitive tissue-culture test should be performed when there is a suspicion of sexually transmitted disease in children, following sexual abuse. The rapid diagnostic tests may be too insensitive to detect organisms in nasopharyngeal or tracheal aspirate for diagnosis of pneumonia, but are recommended for use in conjunctivitis.

Treatment

A topical eye preparation (e.g. tetracycline) can be used in combination with oral erythromycin (50 mg/kg/day in 4 doses for 14 days) in treatment of *Chlamydia ophthalmia*. Erythromycin must be given to reduce the risk of relapse of conjunctivitis when a topical preparation is discontinued, and to prevent development of pneumonia. Erythromycin is used for treatment of pneumonia (dose as above) and there is good evidence that it can be used alone in management of ophthalmia. Children with genital infections should be treated with erythromycin, and adolescents with tetracycline. Parents of infants with neonatal ophthalmia should be investigated and treated in a genito-urinary disease clinic.

Cholera

Notifiable disease

Organism

Widespread epidemic disease is associated only with *Vibrio cholerae* 0-group 1, a Gram-negative motile rod. Other groups may cause severe diarrhoea.

Epidemiology

Since 1961 cholera has spread from India and Southeast Asia to Africa, the Middle East, and even some parts of southern Europe.

Transmission

from an infected person is through contaminated water and food. Shellfish are important vehicles of transmission. With modern sanitation, widespread epidemics are less frequent but may follow natural disasters where there is contamination of food and water and a breakdown of hygiene and sanitation.

Incubation period

is 1–3 days with a range of a few hours to five days. The greater the dose of infecting organisms ingested the shorter the incubation period and the more severe the disease.

Period of infectivity

is variable, and a carrier state may last several months.

Natural history

Illness is characterized by the rapid onset of severe diarrhoea followed by vomiting. Profuse, frequent, and surprisingly painless bowel evacuations accelerate the severe dehydration, shock, and collapse that are the hallmarks of the disease.

Complications of delayed treatment are hypovolaer.iic shock, uncompensated metabolic acidosis, and renal failure, which have a high mortality. However, with improvements in treatment mortality has fallen and should be less than 5 per cent.

Diagnosis

In endemic areas, especially during epidemics, there is no difficulty in diagnosis but sporadic cases will require differentiation from other forms of severe diarrhoea. Diagnosis can be made by microscopic examination of the stool. Culture on bile-salt agar will produce characteristic colonies in 24 hours. The organism can be typed by agglutination with specific antisera. Specific antibody titres can also be measured.

Management

The most important aspect of treatment is the rapid restoration of plasma volume and electrolyte balance. Antibiotics are used for eradication of *Vibrio cholerae* from the gastro-intestinal tract. Co-trimoxazole should be given to children under 10 years of age, and tetracycline to older children (see p. 62 for dosage). The infected child needs to be barrier nursed during the acute phase, and special care taken with handling of stools (enteric precautions—see Glossary) until demonstrated to be non-infectious. Stools of close contacts should be cultured and carriers should be given antibiotics (treatment dose). Attempts must be made to identify the source of infection and appropriate control measures taken.

Cytomegalovirus (CMV)

Organism

Cytomegalovirus (CMV). This is a DNA virus and is a member of the herpes group.

Epidemiology

Up to 50 per cent of individuals have had CMV infection (normally asymptomatic) by childbearing age in industrialized countries. Congenital CMV acquired transplacentally normally follows primary infection in the mother, although reactivation of maternal infection accounts for at least 20 per cent of congenital infections.

Transmission

is from urine, and possibly saliva. The virus can be acquired sexually. Acquired CMV in the newborn may result from transfusion with infected blood or ingestion of infected breast-milk.

Incubation period

is three weeks to three months.

Infectivity

can be prolonged.

Natural history

Congenital infection normally follows an asymptomatic maternal infection at any time during pregnancy. Only about 5 per cent of infected infants develop an acute illness at birth—cytomegalic inclusion disease (CID) associated with petechiae from thrombocytopaenia, hepatitis with jaundice, and microcephaly. Survivors may have features of cerebral palsy. Fewer than 10 per cent of infected infants will present with sensorineural deafness as the only consequence of infection. Acquired neonatal infection in the preterm infant may cause pneumonia and hepatitis, and has a significant mortality in the very low birthweight infant. Infection has occurred following the transfusion of blood from donors infected with CMV. Infection acquired by the term baby, or late in childhood and adolescence is relatively common but usually asymptomatic.

Diagnosis

Diagnosis of congenital CMV is best established by culture of urine or throat swabs within the first two weeks. It is not possible to distinguish between congenital and acquired infection in specimens cultured after this time.

Management and prevention

This is symptomatic as there is no effective antiviral agent. It is important to make an early diagnosis of sensorineural deafness (see rubella management p. 118). No immunization is available. Isolation from other children both within hospital and outside is not indicated and **carriers should not be excluded from nurseries**. There is little evidence that pregnant CMV sero-negative nurses are at increased risk of infection from babies secreting CMV. Nevertheless, nurses and day-care staff should exercise care with the secretions of all their charges and wash their hands after changing nappies. Donor blood for transfusion to the newborn is now routinely tested for CMV antibodies, and when there is evidence of recent infection this is withheld.

Diphtheria

Notifiable disease

Organism

Corynebacterium diphtheriae—a Gram-positive rod.

Epidemiology

The disease is now rare in developed countries because of routine immunization. It still causes considerable morbidity and mortality in the developing countries.

Transmission

is by droplet infection from nose and throat secretions. Unusual sites of infection, for example skin ulcers, may result from direct contact or be spread through fomites (see Glossary).

Incubation period

is 2–5 days but can be longer. Human beings are the only known reservoir of *C. diphtheriae*.

Period of infectivity

is two weeks or less, under four days following antibiotic treatment.

Natural history

The disease usually presents as a membraneous nasopharyngitis or laryngotracheitis. For one to two days a sore throat and low-grade fever are associated with a spreading membrane in the throat that may cause respiratory obstruction (diphtheritic croup) and releases a powerful exotoxin that causes local tissue necrosis and attacks the myocardium of the heart and motor nerves: notably of the soft palate, eyes and diaphragm. The course of the illness depends on the severity of the toxaemia and the degree of immunity conferred by previous immunization. Milder infections in the partially immune may lead to uneventful recovery with the membrane sloughing off in 6–7 days. Severe infections occur in the unimmunized and are characterized by increasing toxaemia progressing to cardio-vascular collapse, stupor, coma, and death.

Diagnosis

Although diptheria is a rare condition in the UK, cases still occur and the diagnosis must be considered in any membraneous condition of the throat, especially in children recently arrived from abroad, or their unimmunized contacts, and in those of doubtful immune status. Cultures should be taken from the nose and throat or from any site which may be contaminated (e.g. weeping skin ulcers). If possible, the swab should be taken from under the membrane. The laboratory should be consulted in advance as special media will be used to accelerate growth and thus identification of the organism.

Management

Children should be isolated and the antitoxin administered immediately the diagnosis is suspected. The dose is calculated according to the size of the membrane, the degree of toxicity, and the duration of illness. Antitoxin may be given im or iv depending on volume required and the severity of illness. Intradermal testing with 1:100 dilution is recommended prior to administration. Benzyl penicillin should be given intravenously. In cases of intermediate severity the potentially lethal complications must be anticipated.

Control measures

Close contacts, whether immunized or not, should have throat swabs, and carriers should be given a course of antibiotic. Contacts previously immunized should receive a booster dose of Diphtheria/ Tetanus/Pertussis (DTP) or DT vaccine if not boosted in the previous five years. Close contacts not previously immunized should be given antibiotic prophylaxis (penicillin or erythromycin) and immunized.

Fifth disease/erythema infectiosum/slapped cheeks syndrome

Organism

Human parvovirus B19—a small DNA virus.

Epidemiology

Infection may occur in any month of the year but peaks occur in late winter, early spring.

Transmission

is by person-to-person spread by droplet infection from the respiratory tract. The virus may also be acquired through infected blood products (e.g. factor VIII concentrates).

Incubation period

is between seven and 22 days.

Infectivity

is high during the early stage of the illness with excretion of the virus from the respiratory tract.

Natural history

Fifth disease is a mild, acute illness occurring most often in children aged 5–14 years. There is a mild prodrome with fever and coryza. The rash is maculopapular and usually starts on the face as a bright red exanthem, hence the term 'slapped cheeks' syndrome. The rash spreads to the trunk and limbs where, on fading, it assumes a lacelike appearance. Constitutional symptoms are minimal: in children, associated respiratory symptoms are the most common feature; in adults, joint pain is a frequent occurrence. The diagnosis in sporadic cases is difficult and not easily differentiated from other exanthemous infections, especially rubella, whereas in community or school outbreaks the clustering of cases results in increased awareness and provides circumstantial support for the diagnosis.

Patients with inherited disorders of red cells can develop aplastic crises following infection with B19 human parvovirus because of temporary arrest of erythropoiesis.

Diagnosis

This is usually a clinical diagnosis. The virus is difficult to identify but serum IgM antibodies can be detected following infection.

Treatment

Symptomatic.

Gastrointestinal infections

Dysentery and typhoid fever are notifiable conditions

Epidemiology

Infections in the UK are normally mild, but may be severe in very young children and the immunosuppressed. Most cases of diarrhoea and vomiting in young children are caused by virus infection: rotavirus, astrovirus, adenovirus, and enterovirus. Bacterial causes of infection include *Salmonella* sp., *Campylobacter jejuni*, and *Yersinia enterocolitica*. *Shigella* sp. and *Vibrio cholerae* infection should be considered in children with severe diarrhoea who have been abroad. Enteropathic *Escherichia coli* infections of infancy are now rarely a cause of disease but outbreaks of verotoxic *E. coli* can cause a severe haemorrhagic colitis in all age groups. Food poisoning may follow ingestion of the exotoxins of *Bacillus cereus* and *Staphylococcus aureus*. The protozoans *Cryptosporidium* and *Giardia lamblia* are increasingly recognized as important causes of diarrhoea, especially in young children. Amoebic dysentery is only seen in children who have been abroad.

Transmission

of all these organisms is by the faecal–oral route, and, for viruses, the respiratory route as well. The incubation period and infectivity are variable (see Appendix 3).

Natural history

Viral infections are normally associated with diarrhoea and vomiting, and sometimes upper-respiratory-tract symptoms. Vomiting may precede diarrhoea in rotavirus infection. These infections are usually self-limiting and recovery occurs in 48–72 hours.

The bacterial infections normally present with diarrhoea and there is generally a systemic 'upset' with fever and headache. Dysentery (bloody, purulent diarrhoea) is a feature of *Shigella* sp. infections, which in young children may be associated with febrile convulsions. *Campylobacter jejuni* infection causes a systemic upset, abdominal pain, and frank blood may be passed in the stool. Similar symptoms may occur with *Yersinia enterocolitica* infection, which may mimic appendicitis or ulcerative colitis. Food poisoning is characterized by vomiting and diarrhoea, with onset a few hours after ingestion of the exotoxin.

Diagnosis

Both vomiting and diarrhoea may be features of other conditions such as meningitis, otitis media, urinary-tract infection, appendicitis, and intussusception. For a fuller discussion see p. 28–9.

In acute florid diarrhoea associated with a systemic illness both stool and blood should be sent for bacterial culture. Even with full investigation in hospital a pathogen is only identified in 80 per cent of cases; while in cases managed in the community the proportion is only 30 per cent. In more chronic diarrhoea, particularly in children, microscopy for ova and cysts becomes more important. Viral identification is possible by electron microscopy; however, this is a time-consuming investigation and consideration has to be given as to whether the result will affect management.

Management

Children with gastroenteritis are at risk of dehydration, and this always needs to be considered in any child with diarrhoea or vomiting. Appropriate treatment depends on an accurate assessment of the degree of dehydration (see Table 7). Children with less than 5 per cent dehydration may be able to remain at home. Those with over 5 per cent dehydration will need hospital admission.

If the diarrhoea is mild and there is no evidence of dehydration, the child can continue on a normal diet at home (breast milk, formula feed, or solids). There is no place at home or in hospital for

Table 7 Signs of different degrees of dehydration

Sign	Less than 5% dehydration	More then 5% dehydration	More than 10% dehydration
Skin	Normal tension	Loss of turgor	Mottled, poor capillary return
Fontanelle (if open)	Normal	Depressed	Deeply depressed
Eyes	Not sunken	Sunken, reduced intraocular pressure	Sunken, reduced intraocular pressure
Lips	Moist	Dry	Dry
Peripheral pulses	Normal	Normal	Poor volume and tachycardia
Blood pressure	Normal	Normal	Low
Behaviour	Unchanged	Lethargic	Prostation, coma
Urine output	Still wetting nappies or urinating at usual frequency	Long periods between micturition	Anuric

NB: Children with hypernatremic dehydration have a doughy feel to the skin and may not appear as dehydrated.

antimotility drugs (opiates, loperamide) in the treatment of acute diarrhoea. Likewise, absorbent mixtures, such as chalk and kaolin, should not be used. Infants and children can become dehydrated quickly, and parents should be warned of the signs of this. Written advice is helpful for parents, advising them to watch for the signs of deterioration, such as worsening diarrhoea or vomiting, decreased frequency of wet nappies/urination, sleepiness, and sunken eyes.

Where vomiting is troublesome, or diarrhoea is more severe, then a glucose electrolyte mixture containing sodium, potassium, chloride, bicarbonate, and glucose in water can be given (80–150 ml/kg/24 h, depending on age). If commercial preparations (Dioralyte, Rehidrat) are prescribed, it is essential to educate parents as to their correct use, to prevent incorrect reconstitution or their being employed as well as, rather than instead of, feeds. Small infants may become hypoglycaemic if such preparations are administered for more than a short period, and the advice of a paediatrician should be sought if no improvement has occurred within 24 hours of the start of the treatment.

In hospital, barrier nursing is required. When a child is less than 5 per cent dehydrated either normal fluid or an electrolyte mixture can be offered. If the child is drinking and dehydration is 5 per cent, an oral glucose electrolyte mixture should be given. If the symptoms fail to respond to oral rehydration, or there is inadequate intake or persistent vomiting, then intravenous rehydration is recommended. In the more severely dehydrated child, intravenous therapy should be started on admission to hospital. Plasma electrolytes must be measured and blood cultures should be collected at the same time. The child is weighed and the amount of fluid to be given is calculated as in Table 8.

Most infants in the UK have isotonic dehydration. If given one-fifth (0.18 per cent) normal saline as fluid replacement, hyponatraemia may develop, so initial rehydration should be with either normal or one-half normal saline with added dextrose to reduce the risk of hypoglycaemia. Hypernatraemic dehydration (plasma sodium more than 150 mmd/l) should be corrected more slowly using normal saline. Antibiotics may sometimes be given to treat systemic illness and shorten the period of infectivity, as shown in Table 8.

Post-enteritis syndrome

This is characterized by continuing diarrhoea and is often associated with lactose intolerance, which can be diagnosed by testing the liquid portion of the stool for reducing sugars using Clinitest tablets (a value over 1 per cent is significant). Cows' milk protein intoler-

Table 8 Treatment of dehydration

Example: a 10 kg infant with 10% dehydration—

(1) Treat shock with plasma:
     20 ml/kg over first half hour = 200 ml

(2) Fluid deficit = 1 kg = 1000 ml
     Aim to correct half deficit in first 8 hours, and half in next 16 hours:

     First 8 hours: $\frac{500}{8}$ ml = 62 ml/h, then $\frac{500}{16}$ ml = 31 ml/h

(3) Aim to give maintenance fluid, i.e. 10 kg infant requires
     100 ml/kg/day, so needs:

     $\frac{1000}{24}$ = 43 ml/h

Thus, in first half hour, 200 ml plasma, then 105 ml (62 + 43)/h to
8 hours, and 74 ml (31 + 43)/h from 8–24 hours

---

ance may also develop. For both conditions a lactose-free soya milk
(Cow & Gate formula S, Prosobee, Wysoy) may be prescribed by the
paediatrician.

GUIDELINES FOR PREVENTION OF GASTROENTERITIS IN DAY-CARE FACILITIES, SCHOOLS, AND THE HOME

Special attention should be given to the following.

1. In making up formula feeds care must be taken that bottles are
    adequately sterilized and milk is not allowed to stand for long
    periods.

2. Ensure everyone (staff, parents, and children) understands the
    importance of handwashing with soap and hot water after using

Diseases

Table 9 Antibiotics given for specific gastrointestinal infections

Infection	Antibiotics
Campylobacter jejuni	In severe infection only, erythromycin 30 mg/kg/day, 3 times daily for 3 days
Entamoeba histolytica	Metronidazole 50 mg/kg/day 3 times daily for 5 days
Giardia lamblia	Metronidazole 15 mg/kg/day, 3 doses daily for 5 days
Salmonella typhi	Chloramphenicol 50 mg/kg/day oral, or 75 mg/kg/day iv, 4 times daily for 14 days; or ampicillin 100 mg/kg/day, 4 times daily for 14 days
Shigella dysentery	Ampicillin 100 mg/kg/day in 4 doses daily for 5 days, or co-trimoxazole 10 mg/kg/day as trimethoprin in 2 divided doses for 5 days
Vibrio cholerae	In children aged nine and under, co-trimoxazole as for Shigella; in children aged 10 and over, tetracycline 50 mg/kg/day 4 times daily for 2 days

the toilet, changing nappies, and before preparing or eating food.

3. Toileting and nappy-changing areas must be well separated from food-preparation areas.

4. Where cases have occurred, children and staff with acute diarrhoea should be excluded for the duration of symptoms where no organism is identified. Where a specific cause is identified, negative stool samples may need to be obtained before readmission (see Table 10). Exclusion may not always be necessary in schools where effective hygiene practices can be implemented. Decisions will depend on the organism and local facilities, and will be made in consultation with the designated medical officer.

5. Specimens may need to be taken from contacts of cases. However, the Medical Officer of Environmental Health

Table 10   A guide to exclusion of children from day care or school following gastroenteritis. Children should be excluded while symptomatic, although exclusion may be less strictly observed for secondary-school children. (Adapted from: *Notes on the control of human sources of gastrointestinal infections, infestation and bacterial intoxication in the United Kingdom.* Communicable Disease Report, Supplement 1, 1983.)

Organism	Criteria of clearance	Notifiable
Campylobacter	When diarrhoea ceases	No
Bacillary dysentery (Shigellosis)	3 negative faeces at least 24 hrs apart	Yes
Amoebic dysentery	3 negative faeces (for cysts)	Yes
E. coli (enteropathogenic strains)	3 negative faeces	No
Virus gastroenteritis Rotavirus Others	When diarrhoea ceases	No
Salmonellosis (excluding typhoid, paratyphoid)	3 negative faeces	Yes
Typhoid, paratyphoid	3 negative faeces	Yes
Giardiasis	None	No

(MOEH) will need to give advice as to when this is appropriate.

6. Where there is a sudden outbreak involving several children, food poisoning must be considered and the MOEH involved immediately.

7. It will need to be explained to staff that most cases of childhood diarrhoea have a viral cause and stool cultures will be negative.

Glandular fever (infectious mononucleosis)

Organism
Epstein–Barr virus (EBV) which is a herpes virus.

Epidemiology
Infection is often subclinical in infancy and childhood, but commonly produces illness in the adolescent and young adult, and most adults are seropositive, indicating that they have experienced a previous infection.

Transmission
is by saliva, with spread by close contact in young children. Glandular fever has been dubbed 'the kissing disease' because of the high incidence of clinical infection in late adolescence. Reactivation of EBV infection may occur in the immunosuppressed patient.

Incubation period
is between 30 and 50 days.

Infectivity
may be prolonged for several months following infection.

Natural history
The illness normally begins with fever, headache, and malaise, and is followed by a severe sore throat and lymphadenopathy. Fever may last from several days to two weeks. Lymphadenopathy is generalized but more pronounced in the glands of the neck. A white exudate is often present on the enlarged tonsils and petechiae may

be seen on the palate. An erythematous maculo-papular rash is seen frequently in children given ampicillin inappropriately for treatment of this infection. Splenomegaly can be detected in most patients and liver enlargement, sometimes associated with jaundice, although common, is a less consistent clinical finding. Uncommon complications include pneumonia, aseptic meningitis, and transverse myelitis. Pneumonia is a feature of EBV infection in children with AIDS.

Diagnosis

When tonsillitis, lymphadenopathy, and splenomegaly are seen together, infectious mononucleosis is the probable diagnosis. A rash developing after ampicillin prescribed for tonsillitis is often diagnostic of EBV infection.

Haematological changes in infectious mononucleosis are non-specific; there may be a leukopenia or a leucocytosis but there is normally an increase in 'atypical' lymphocytes. Patients develop a high titre of specific antibodies known as agglutinins because of their ability to cause sheep red blood cells to clump together. These are detected in the 'monospot' or 'Paul Bunnell' tests. However, these may not become positive until 3–4 weeks after the onset of symptoms.

Other conditions to be differentiated from infectious mononucleosis include streptococcal tonsillitis, diphtheria, viral hepatitis, and acquired cytomegalovirus infection. If recovery is delayed, it is important to exclude acute lymphoblastic leukaemia which may present with similar signs.

Treatment

This is symptomatic with analgesics and antipyretics. Indications for hospital admission include airway obstruction from large tonsils (more common in the young adult than child) or neurological complications. Isolation is not required and there is no quarantine period.

Gonococcal infections

Ophthalmia neonatorum is a notifiable disease

Organism

Neisseria gonorrhoeae which is a paired, Gram-negative coccus.

Epidemiology

This infection occurs only in humans. It is commonest amongst adults with multiple sexual partners.

Transmission

is by direct sexual contact, or to the infant during parturition causing ophthalmia neonatorum (a purulent discharge from the eye of an infant within 21 days of birth). Infection during childhood is almost certainly the result of sexual abuse, and cannot occur through other ways such as contact with an adult in a bath, from lavatory seats, or towels.

Incubation period

is 2–7 days.

Infectivity

continues until the disease is treated.

Natural history

Gonococcal ophthalmia neonatorum in the newborn normally develops as an acute purulent conjunctivitis 2–5 days after birth. Untreated, corneal scarring or even loss of the eye may follow. Spread to the joints or meninges may occur. Neonatal vaginitis has been reported but is rare. Infection in childhood may result in vulvovaginitis or urethritis, and after puberty in endocervicitis or pelvic inflammatory disease. Proctitis, pharyngitis or conjunctivitis may be seen in all age groups.

Diagnosis

A Gram stain of the exudate should be performed immediately in the presence of purulent conjunctivitis. In many laboratories this is performed on a smear taken from a single swab which is also used for culture. Gonococcal culture is indicated following sexual abuse or in a child with a vaginal or urethral discharge (see Table 3). *Chlamydia trachomatis* infection may produce similar symptoms in childhood. A serological test for syphilis should be considered where gonococcal infection is present.

Treatment

Treatment of ophthalmia neonatorum with systemic benzyl penicillin and saline washes to the eye should be started immediately following identification of Gram-negative cocci on Gram stain, or culture of *Neisseria gonorrhoeae*. In childhood gonococcal infection, a single injection of procaine penicillin, or oral ampicillin can be used. Amoxicillin and ampicillin are ineffective for anorectal infections and pharyngitis. Adolescents should also be treated with procaine penicillin. Penicillin resistance is unusual; children with a true penicillin allergy should be treated with spectinomycin and erythromycin. In neonatal infections the mother and father or consort should be referred to a genitourinary disease clinic. In older children, the local procedure for suspected sexual abuse must be initiated.

Haemolytic uraemic syndrome

This syndrome is relatively uncommon even in specialized hospital practice. However, its inclusion in this book is justified by the importance of early recognition and the apparent increase in incidence reflected in reports to the British Paediatric Surveillance Unit (BPSU). It is now the commonest cause of acute renal failure in childhood.

Organism

The exact cause is unknown. The occurrence of mini-epidemics suggests an infection but to date no organism has been identified consistently. Current interest is focused on verotoxin-producing *Escherichia coli* but the syndrome has been associated with many other viruses and bacteria.

Epidemiology

There are small outbreaks but most cases occur sporadically. There can be a familial or genetic predisposition, with both autosomal recessive and dominant forms reported. The syndrome predominates in children under three years of age, has a mortality of 20 per cent, and there is significant chronic illness in some survivors.

Natural history

There is usually a well-defined prodromal illness such as gastroenteritis often with bloody diarrhoea. Fever is transient and mild but the child looks and feels ill with quite severe abdominal pain that may lead to referral to a surgical ward. Although the gastrointestinal symptoms and signs may settle after one or two days, the child's general condition remains poor and more specific features of the syndrome develop: haematuria and proteinuria with oliguria which may progress rapidly to anuria; hypertension; haemolytic anaemia with red-cell fragmentation and thrombocytopaenia prominent on a blood film; CNS signs such as alterations in consciousness and seizure activity.

The histo-pathological lesion is a widespread thrombotic micro-angiopathy with endothelial damage resulting either directly from a toxic agent or indirectly through mechanical interference with the microcirculation from fibrin deposition. In addition to the anaemia and thrombocytopaenia described above, plasma urea and creatinine are elevated. Depending on the stage of the illness there may be a decrease in clotting factors and an increase in fibrin-degradation products.

Management

As this syndrome has a significant mortality, intensive treatment should be started as soon as the condition is suspected. This is best achieved with specialized staff and facilities and frequent monitoring of vital signs, fluid and electrolyte balance, body weight, blood pressure, and the early provision of peritoneal dialysis. Severe anaemia should be corrected by small transfusions of packed cells. Over-hydration is particularly dangerous and management is aided by establishing a central venous line. Broad-spectrum antibiotics, but not those potentially nephrotoxic, are usually given in the early stages of the syndrome as the presenting features are difficult to distinguish from those of severe infection, but there is no evidence that they are always necessay. Steroids are not indicated.

Although milder cases with oliguria may resolve spontaneously without dialysis, there is evidence that the early introduction of peritoneal dialysis may improve the outcome. Haemodialysis is rarely necessary but peritoneal dialysis may be required for several weeks before the gradual return of renal function. In survivors the majority of children go on to complete recovery, although, in a few there may be some residual renal insufficiency or hypertension.

Haemophilus influenzae infection

Organism

Haemophilus influenzae is a small, Gram-negative cocco-bacillus classified into capsular serotypes a–f and those without capsules.

Epidemiology

Haemophilus influenzae inhabits the upper respiratory tract and asymptomatic colonization is common with non-capsulated strains present in the throat of 60–90 per cent of individuals, and encapsulated strains in approximately 5 per cent. Most *H. influenzae* meningitis in the newborn is caused by non-typeable organisms; *H. influenzae* serotype b produces epiglottitis and meningitis in later infancy and childhood, with infection uncommon over the age of five. Outside the neonatal period, the non-typeable strains cause less severe illness, such as otitis media.

Transmission

is by inhalation of droplets of respiratory-tract secretions containing the organisms.

Incubation period

is not known, and difficult to establish because children may become colonized for some time before infection occurs.

Natural history

H. influenzae, is a major cause of meningitis from the neonatal period to the age of four. Epiglottitis is invariably caused by this organism and is most common from two to four years but can occur during later childhood and adult life (see p. 000). *H. influenzae* is also a cause of septic arthritis, cellulitis, bacteraemia, pneumonia, and empyema.

Diagnosis

For invasive infections, appropriate body fluids such as CSF, blood, or synovial fluid should be obtained for Gram stain and culture. Antigen detection in body fluids using latex agglutination or counter immunoelectrophoresis tests may be useful, especially in children who have received prior antibiotic treatment.

Management

Invasive infections such as meningitis and epiglottitis in infants and children over one month of age should be treated with ampicillin and chloramphenicol. For the neonate, ampicillin and an aminoglycoside or cephalosporin (e.g. cefotaxime) can be used. A single antimicrobial can be given once the results of sensitivity testing is available. Up to 10 per cent of invasive strains are resistant to ampicillin; chloramphenicol resistance is rare. It is recommended that a minimum of 10 days' treatment is given. Localized infections such as otitis media can usually be successfully treated with ampicillin but, in the case of resistant strains, alternative antibiotics include co-trimoxazole, clavulanic acid, or cephaclor.

Chemoprophylaxis

When there is another pre-school child in the house of a case of invasive type b infection, rifampicin prophylaxis is recommended for all household contacts. The index case should also receive rifampicin, since standard treatment does not eradicate nasopharyngeal carriage. Rifampicin is an enzyme inducer in the liver, and chloramphenicol plasma levels are lowered when both antibiotics are given together. Because of this it is advisable to give rifampicin towards the end of the course of treatment.

Prospects for immunization

A vaccine consisting of purified type b capsular polysaccharide is safe and effective in preventing invasive type b infections, but only in children of 24 months or older. This vaccine is recommended as a routine immunization in the USA where *H. influenzae* is more common, but is **not licensed for use in the UK**. Another vaccine which combines a polysaccharide and protein antigen appears to be more effective and is undergoing evaluation at present.

Hand, foot, and mouth disease

Organism

Coxsackie virus—several different sub-types.

Epidemiology

This is a relatively common condition which tends to occur in epidemics and is not to be confused with foot-and-mouth disease which occurs in cattle. Infections predominate in the summer and autumn in pre-school children.

Transmission

is by droplets from the respiratory tract, by direct contact with the rash and by the faecal–oral route.

Incubation period

is 3–5 days.

Infectivity

can be prolonged as the virus may remain in the stool for several weeks.

Natural history

The illness is characterized by vesicular lesions with a red base, which in the oral cavity are seen on the fauces, tongue, and side of the mouth. The rash is also seen on the hands and soles of the feet. There may be a history of low-grade fever for 4–6 days preceding the rash.

Diagnosis

This is on clinical grounds. Viral isolation is unnecessary.

Management

No treatment is needed. Because of the ease of spread amongst pre-school children they should be kept away from their peers until the lesions clear from the hands.

Hepatitis A (infective jaundice)

Notifiable disease

Organism

An enterovirus type 72.

Epidemiology

This is the commonest cause of jaundice in children.

Transmission

is via the faecal–oral route and also occurs through contamination of food or water as the virus is relatively resistant. Epidemics result from contamination with raw sewage. In children the disease is relatively mild with anicteric infection being common (approximately 80 per cent).

Incubation period

is 15–40 days.

Infectivity

is maximal during the latter half of the incubation period but disappears in the few days following development of jaundice or other symptoms. Infection is commoner amongst children in poor social circumstances and in institutional care or other circumstances where hygiene or sanitation are poor.

Natural history

In symptomatic cases fever commonly precedes the onset of jaundice and is accompanied (with or without jaundice) by headache, anorexia, nausea, vomiting, and abdominal pain from a tender, enlarged liver. Once jaundice accompanied by dark urine appears the child may feel better, although return of appetite and full vigour is usually delayed until clearing of the jaundice in about two weeks. Convalescence is brief and full recovery the usual outcome. Extremely rarely a child may develop liver failure from fulminating hepatitis.

Diagnosis

Diagnosis is usually on clinical grounds. Urobilinogen can be detected in the urine at the onset of jaundice. Laboratory tests show a transient rise in serum transaminase levels for 1–3 weeks with a rise in bilirubin at the peak of transaminase disturbance. When the course of the illness appears to be more severe or prolonged than expected, hepatitis B infection should be excluded (see p. 77–79). Serological tests for IgG anti-HAV (hepatitis A virus) and IgM anti-HAV are available but rarely indicated.

Management

There is no specific treatment. Hospital admission is undesirable and rarely necessary. However, if this is unavoidable, the child should be nursed in a cubicle and enteric precautions taken (see Glossary). The importance of personal hygiene in preventing spread should be emphasized to parents and other carers of children. Careful handwashing is essential after nappy-changing or toiletting and before preparing or serving food and drink. Children with undiagnosed jaundice should be managed with precautions applicable to both hepatitis A and B until a diagnosis is made. This means treating blood and body fluids as if hepatitis B positive. Close contacts can be given human normal immunoglobulin (HNIG): 250 mg for children up to the age of nine; 500 mg for children of 10 and over.

Hepatitis B

Notifiable disease

Organism

A DNA-containing virus 42 nm in diameter. The virus is a double-shelled particle with the outer surface component, the hepatitis B surface antigen (HBsAg) used as the marker which identifies the carrier state or chronic hepatitis B. Two other antigens of hepatitis B infection have also been identified - the core antigen (HBcAg) and the e antigen (HBeAg), the latter being used as a marker of infectivity. The disease is transmitted by the introduction through the skin or mucous membrane of blood or blood products containing the virus.

Epidemiology

Children at particular risk include those who receive frequent transfusions of blood or blood products, e.g. in haemophilia; those on chronic haemo-dialysis; infants born to mothers who are HBeAg positive and, to a lesser extent, those with mothers who are HBsAg positive without being 'e' positive. Because the prevalence of the carrier state varies so much according to racial group, the risk of perinatal transmission will also vary with ethnic origin. In Asia the risk to infants born to mothers of Chinese origin may be as high as 40 per cent, whereas in Caucasian mothers the carrier state is uncommon (0.1–0.2 per cent) and therefore perinatal transmission is extremely rare. It is, however, important to identify intravenous drug abusing mothers as a high-risk group. The virus does not cross the placenta and transmission from mother to child probably occurs during or just after birth from a leak of maternal blood into the infant's circulation or through a break in the skin or mucous membranes. Subclinical infection with the development of a chronic carrier state may occur in the child. There is a clear association between the carrier state, chronic liver disease, and the development of hepato-cellular carcinoma in later life, particularly in non-Caucasians.

Incubation period

is usually 60–90 days but may be as long as six months.

Infectivity

is low unless there is blood-to-blood contact.

Natural history

Infection with hepatitis B virus usually results in an apparently mild illness with anorexia, nausea, and general malaise. A prodrome with arthralgia and a rash may occur. Obvious jaundice can develop but, as with hepatitis A, anicteric infection is common. Marked jaundice is unusual in children, although the serum bilirubin is usually elevated. Compared with hepatitis A, laboratory testing reveals a more prolonged disturbance of serum transaminases, usually for 30–60 days. Fulminant hepatitis occasionally occurs with onset of hepatic failure within four weeks after the onset of acute hepatitis. As with hepatitis A, the overall prognosis including the survival rate is influenced by age, being much better in children than in adults.

Hepatitis B is also associated with more lasting morbidity and about 10 per cent will develop evidence of chronic disease, either chronic persistent hepatitis or chronic active hepatitis. The chronic state may follow mild anicteric forms of hepatitis. Primary liver carcinoma is an established consequence in young adults following childhood infection, though this is commoner amongst individuals infected in Africa or Asia rather than in Europe.

Diagnosis

Serological testing for HBsAg is useful in diagnosis and for the detection of carriers. The presence of HBeAg indicates that an individual will be infectious, but if HBe antibody is also present, the infectivity will be low.

Management

There is no specific treatment for hepatitis B infection. As for hepatitis A, mild cases should be cared for in the home. Where hospitalization is required, infected children should be barrier nursed and precautions taken in handling blood and other body fluids. Patients with undiagnosed jaundice should be managed with precautions applicable to both hepatitis A and B until the aetiology is established. Infants born to HBsAg positive mothers do not need to be isolated but care should be taken with blood/body fluids because 1–2 per cent will have become infected by perinatal transmission. They may require immunization, particularly if the mother is e antigen positive (see p. 193). Gloves should be worn by staff undertaking procedures involving the handling of blood or body fluids of these patients.

Herpes simplex

Organism

This is a DNA virus. Type 1 (HSV1) is a cause of cold sores and encephalitis in childhood, and type 2 (HSV2) is the cause of most neonatal infection.

NEONATAL INFECTION

Epidemiology

This occurs in approximately one per 50 000 live births. Most cases are associated with primary infection of the genital tract with HSV2.

Transmission

is by a maternal viraemia, by an ascending route to the uterus or during passage down the birth canal. The risk of infection following vaginal delivery in the presence of primary infection in the mother is about 50 per cent, but less than 8 per cent for recurrent infection.

Infectivity

is low (see Management).

Natural history

Infection may present as a generalized systemic illness with hepatitis and encephalitis; as localized central nervous system disease; or as localized infection of the skin, eyes, or mouth. The mortality is high with systemic disease.

Diagnosis

This is by tissue culture of secretions but a positive result may take three days. Rapid techniques using direct fluorescent antibody are being developed at present. Serology has no place in the diagnosis of acute infection.

Prevention and management

Because most cases result from a primary maternal infection where the history is short, diagnosis and treatment in the newborn are often delayed until many hours after onset of symptoms. It is current practice to perform regular viral culture on genital-tract secretions in women with known HSV infection during the last few weeks of pregnancy, so that Caesarean section can be undertaken early in labour if genital lesions are present. However, because of the delay in obtaining positive cultures and since most neonatal infection follows undiagnosed infection in the mother, this practice is of limited usefulness.

HSV infection in the new-born is treated with acyclovir; morbidity and mortality are reduced by treatment, in both neurological and generalized disease. Many paediatricians recommend treatment of all infants born to mothers with primary infection. Because of the low risk in association with recurrent maternal infection, it is recommended that infants born to such mothers are observed for at least 10 days after delivery and only treated when symptomatic.

The infected mother can nurse her own baby but needs to be kept in isolation from other infants. Because the risk of infection from attendants is extremely low, nurses with cold sores should be allowed to work provided lesions are covered and scrupulous attention is paid to handwashing.

CHILDHOOD INFECTION

Epidemiology

Infections are common in childhood but most are minor.

Transmission

is by direct spread from saliva.

Incubation period

is 2–12 days.

Infectivity

following primary HSV1 can be prolonged for several weeks.

Natural history

Gingivostomatitis (infection of the gums and mouth) is the commonest significant manifestation of type 1 infection, presenting with fever and painful vesicles in the affected area. Infections in children with eczema may result in Kaposi's varicelliform eruption (eczema herpeticum) which may be complicated by bacterial infection. The lesions are similar to those seen in zoster (shingles) but are not restricted to the dermatome distribution (see Glossary). Where herpetic lesions are seen in the genital tract in childhood, they are almost certainly the result of sexual abuse and usually are due to HSV2. Encephalitis results from HSV type 1 and is usually a primary infection; it presents with altered consciousness and convulsions, and has a 50 per cent mortality.

Diagnosis

Because of the serious nature of both eczema herpeticum and encephalitis, a clinical diagnosis is sufficient for treatment to be started. The virus can be identified in tissue culture, by electron microscopy; rapid diagnostic methods are being introduced. Only rarely is virus isolated from the CSF in encephalitis.

Treatment

The systemic antiviral agent, acyclovir, is the treatment of choice and should be given without delay in severe infections.

Influenza

Organism

The influenza viruses are orthomyxoviruses of three antigenic types (A, B, and C) but epidemic disease is caused by types A and B. In contrast to most other viruses, influenza A and B (especially A) constantly alter their antigenic substructure—antigenic 'drift'. This limits the effectiveness of vaccines from year to year and these have to be frequently modified to fit the components of the prevalent strains.

Epidemiology

The highest attack rates occur in school-age children, with secondary spread to adults and younger children in the household. Attack rates depend on the immunity conferred by previous infections or immunization. New strains occurring through antigenic drift may cause widespread epidemics which occur particularly in the winter, lasting 1–2 months.

Transmission

is by airborne droplets and through articles such as handkerchiefs recently contaminated by nasopharyngeal secretions.

Incubation period

is 1–3 days.

Infectivity

is high for 24 hours before symptoms appear, and for 24–48 hours thereafter.

Natural history

There is a wide spectrum of severity. Rapid onset of fever with rigors is accompanied by headache, diffuse muscle aches, and a dry cough. More widespread signs of respiratory infection may then follow including nasal congestion, a painful throat, stridor, and signs of lower-respiratory-tract involvement, including pneumonia, which is particularly likely to develop in children suffering from chronic cardiac or respiratory disease. In young infants influenza may mimic generalized sepsis with relatively few localizing respiratory signs. Although influenza alone can produce a severe respiratory illness, secondary bacterial invasion of the lungs with such organisms as *Staphylococcus aureus* and *Klebsiella pneumoniae* is particularly dangerous. Otitis media is another common bacterial complication. Viral complications such as myocarditis and encephalitis are seen in adults but are rarely a problem in childhood.

Diagnosis

Rapid diagnosis is rarely necessary but is possible through identification of the influenza antigen in nasopharyngeal secretions by immunofluorescent techniques or enzyme-linked immunosorbent assay (ELISA). Serological diagnosis is possible retrospectively by demonstrating a rise in antibody between acute and convalescent sera.

Treatment

Treatment is symptomatic in previously healthy individuals.

Control measures

It is recommended that children of all ages with cystic fibrosis should be immunized annually against the prevalent strain. Similarly, immunization should be considered for other children who may be at risk of severe infection, such as those with chronic lung and heart diseases.

Kawasaki disease (mucocutaneous lymph node syndrome (MCNLS))

Report to British Paediatric Surveillance Unit (BPSU)

Organism

Unknown. An infectious agent is suspected but none has been identified consistently to date.

Epidemiology

First described in Japan (1967) where the incidence is particularly high at about one in every 1000 children. The disease is now recognized world-wide. Over 100 cases were reported in 1987 to the BPSU but under-diagnosis and under-reporting remain. The vast majority of cases occur in children under five years with a peak occurrence at 1–2 years. The male : female ratio is 1.6 : 1.

Transmission

is unknown but even close childhood contacts do not seem to be at any increased risk.

Natural history

The illness begins with an abrupt onset of fever which may persist for 5–15 days, or even longer in some cases, and is unresponsive to antibiotics. After 2–3 days of unexplained fever, the characteristic features of the disease develop in succession and should suggest the diagnosis. These are:

(1) red eyes from inflamed conjunctivae;

(2)   changes in the mouth—red, swollen lips which progress to cracking and fissuring after several days, strawberry tongue, pharyngeal erythema;

(3)   rash: generalized erythematous eruption which may be punctate or maculo-papular;

(4)   cervical lymphadenopathy—non-suppurative and may be unilateral;

(5)   changes in fingers and toes—reddening, oedema, with desquamation on the tips after 2–3 weeks.

Resolution of fever with obvious improvement in the child's condition may have occurred by the time desquamation occurs, but fretfulness and anorexia may persist for several weeks. Other features in some patients include diarrhoea, arthritis, and arthralgia; aseptic meningitis, pneumonia, and a sterile pyuria. The most worrying feature of Kawasaki disease is occasional cardiac and coronary artery involvement. Routine echo-cardiography or angiography have demonstrated abnormalities of the coronary arteries ranging from mild dilatation or tortuosity to aneurysm formation in about 20 per cent of patients. Aneurysms are particularly frequent under the age of six months and may first appear 2–3 weeks after the onset of the illness. They usually regress but there is a mortality rate of 1–2 per cent usually from coronary artery thrombosis with myocardial infarction. Although there may be ECG changes (e.g. lengthening of QT_c interval, T-wave flattening, and depression of S-T segments) aneurysm formation can occur without any ECG abnormality.

Diagnosis

There is no specific test for Kawasaki disease. Diagnosis is based on the complex of characteristic clinical and laboratory features occurring after several days of unexplained fever. The most useful test findings are a thrombocytosis of over 450 000 and often exceeding 1 000 000 mm³ by the second or third week of the disease; a raised erythrocyte sedimentation rate (ESR), a leucocytosis of over 15 000 mm³; elevated C-reactive protein and alpha-2 globulin. Many other diseases produce rashes, mucocutaneous lesions, and lymphadeno-pathy, but rarely as many as four of the five characteristic clinical features described above. Frequently confused with Kawasaki disease, especially in the first few days of the illness, are measles, scarlet fever, glandular fever, roseola infantum, and the systemic form of juvenile chronic arthritis (Still's disease).

Management

Isolation is unnecessary. With the possible exception of immuno-globulin (see below) there is no specific treatment which can prevent the potentially serious complications such as coronary artery involvement, carditis, and arthritis. Aspirin has been shown to reduce the risk of complications. It is administered initially in anti-inflammatory doses of 80–100 mg/kg/day in four divided doses. Once the fever has settled, the dose is reduced to 5 mg/day in one dose in order to decrease platelet adhesiveness. Low-dose aspirin treatment is continued for at least three months. If an aneurysm has been detected, aspirin therapy is recommended until the aneurysm resolves, which may take many months. It has been suggested that intravenous immunoglobulin given in the acute phase of the illness may be helpful in preventing aneurysm formation, but this needs to be confirmed. Corticosteroid drugs are contraindicated.

Malaria

Notifiable disease

Organism

Plasmodium species (*falciparum, ovale, vivax, malariae*)—a proto-zoan.

Epidemiology

Imported malaria has increased dramatically in the seventies and eighties (Fig. 3); between 200 and 300 cases in children under 16 are now notified annually in England and Wales. The disease is endemic in Africa (except on the Mediterranean coast), the Indian subcontinent (ISC), the tropical Far East, South and Central America but not the West Indian Islands (except Haiti). Over half the UK cases are now travellers from the ISC (mainly vivax malaria) but there has been a recent upsurge in those from Africa (mainly the more serious falciparum variety).

Transmission

is by the *Anopheles* mosquito and does not occur within the UK.

Incubation period

is 6–16 days, depending on the species; because the symptoms can be mild the child may present months after leaving the endemic area.

Natural history

The infected child typically has an intermittent fever with rigors and sweats which may occasionally progress to a convulsion and neurological involvement (cerebral malaria). Late and persistent symptoms are less common in children but do occur; they include

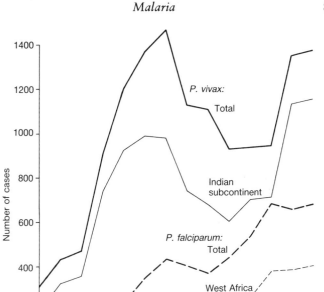

Fig. 3 Malaria, UK 1973–86.

nausea, jaundice, arthralgia, abdominal and back pain. Signs of malaria in infants may be non-specific with loss of appetite, irritability, and lethargy. Where infection has been frequent the child may be anaemic with splenomegaly. Congenital infection has been seen in the UK, usually amongst mothers born in the UK who have visited endemic areas.

Diagnosis

This is by a thick blood film which requires a fresh specimen sent promptly (with warning) to an experienced person. If anti-malarials have been taken, these must be specified along with the country of travel.

Management

Uncomplicated attacks can be treated with chloroquine. When *P. falciparum* acquired in areas of chloroquine resistance is a possibility, specialist advice should be obtained. Children with cerebral malaria, which has a high mortality, should be treated by physicians with experience of this disease.

Prevention is better than cure. For protection when travelling abroad see p. 270–5.

Measles

Notifiable disease

Organism

Measles virus, an RNA-containing virus in the paramyxovirus family.

Epidemiology

Because immunization falls short of targets in the UK, this disease is both endemic and epidemic (Fig. 4). It is uncommon under the age of one because of protection from maternal antibody. The peak incidence is at school entry when infection is almost completely confined to unimmunized children. In the decade 1976–85, 165 children died from measles in the UK.

Transmission

is by airborne droplet spread (coughing and sneezing), from freshly soiled handkerchiefs, or by direct contact.

Incubation period

is 10 days (range 8–13).

Infectivity

is high. Children are infectious from shortly before the first symptoms to four days after the rash appears. They are most infectious prior to the appearance of the rash. In a highly susceptible population one case will, on average, cause 15 others. In a school this can mean 30–40 per cent of unimmunized children, in the home 70 per cent.

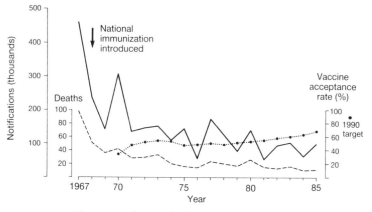

Fig. 4 Measles, England and Wales 1967–85.

Natural history

Initially, the child develops coryzal symptoms which are followed by conjunctivitis causing photophobia and a dry cough. The tonsils may be red and Koplik's spots (like grains of salt) appear on the inside of the cheeks beside the molar teeth. After 2–3 days the temperature peaks and the rash appears first behind the ears then spreading over the face and down the body. The rash is more confluent over the upper part of the body. (For timing of signs see Fig. 2, p. 15.) Koplik's spots fade on the fifth or sixth day. If complications do not occur the temperature also returns to normal and the child feels better, though the cough may persist for another week. Most school-age children will, on average, miss a week of school with measles.

Complications are common and include croup in the prodromal period, viral or bacterial pneumonia, otitis media and conductive deafness, enteritis, encephalopathy, fits, and more severe CNS disease which can be fatal or cause brain damage. A late complication is subacute sclerosing panencephalitis (SSPE) occurring 5–10 years after infection. This is a slow, untreatable degenerative disease of the nervous system which is always handicapping and fatal in approximately 50 per cent of cases. The rate of complications of any kind amongst notified cases of measles is 1 in 10, while 1 in 70 children with the disease are admitted to hospital. Encephalopathy (including fits) occurs in 1 case in 500, and death in 1 case in 5000. Measles is also the most important cause of severe morbidity and mortality in immunosuppressed children being treated for malignant disease.

Diagnosis

Diagnosis is based on history and clinical signs. Many other rashes may be incorrectly diagnosed as measles unless the whole pattern of symptoms is considered.

Management

The child with uncomplicated disease needs nursing and temperature control rather than medication, other than paracetamol. It is traditional to darken the room, but most children will simply turn away from the light. Complications should be treated appropriately. Admission to hospital should be avoided where possible because of the risk to immunosuppressed children. There is no place for antibiotics unless there is clear evidence of bacterial infection, which, if it occurs, takes place late in the course of the disease.

Control measures

1. Isolation. This is indicated for four days after the appearance of the rash. The risk to immunosuppressed children should be considered (see p. 258).
2. Immunization (see p. 200–5). If live measles virus vaccine is given within 72 hours of exposure, it may lessen the disease in that child.
3. Immune globulin. This will prevent or modify measles in susceptible children if given within three days of exposure (0.25 ml/kg im). The dose should be double for immunosuppressed children (0.5 ml/kg) up to a maximum of 15 ml. A preparation of human measles immunoglobulin with a higher concentration of measles

antibody is available in Scotland (Scottish National Blood Transfusion Service).

Family education

Many of the public and even some members of the nursing and medical profession believe that measles is a trivial illness. This has led to inadequate vaccine uptake and allowed disproportionate concern about vaccine reactions. A useful health-education device is the description by the author Roald Dahl of his daughter Olivia's death from measles. It is available in written form by sending a stamped addressed envelope to: Sandwell Health Authority, 8 Grange Road, West Bromwich, West Midlands B70 8PD.

Meningococcal disease

Meningitis is a notifiable condition

Organism

Neisseria meningitidis is a Gram-negative diplococcus. There are nine serotypes (A, B, C, D, X, Y, Z, 29-E, and W-135). Groups B and C are currently the most prevalent in the UK.

Epidemiology

Trends in the occurrence of meningococcal disease have shown periodic upsurges (e.g. 1940–5, the mid-seventies, and 1986–8.) *N. meningitidis* is currently the commonest cause of bacterial meningitis among children in the UK, mostly in the pre-school population. In 1986 there were 582 notified cases of meningococcal meningitis among children in England and Wales.

Transmission

occurs from person to person from naso-pharyngeal droplets or respiratory secretions. Infection may also develop in children and adults who have been carriers, and they may spread the disease, particularly to their close contacts.

Incubation period

is variable because infection may follow colonization. Treatment of invasive disease does not always result in eradication of the organism from the nasopharynx.

Natural history

The reasons why this organism suddenly invades a particular individual are not well understood. Onset of meningococcal bacteraemia or meningitis may be abrupt, with fever, rigors, and prostration. A petechial rash (sometimes preceded by a maculo-papular rash) progressing to widespread and extensive bleeding into the skin (purpura) is characteristic of the more severe cases in which death may occur within a few hours. In convalescence, the purpuric lesions may slough (purpura necrotica). Pneumonia, unsuspected bacteraemia, arthritis, infective endocarditis, and chronic meningococcaemia are other less common invasive infections caused by this organism. Disease occurs at all ages but is most common in children under five years of age.

Diagnosis

Cultures of blood and cerebrospinal fluid are most useful in establishing the diagnosis. The organism may also be cultured from skin lesions and, rarely, synovial fluid. Rapid diagnosis may also be afforded through latex-agglutination tests which detect group-specific antigens in body fluids (e.g. CSF, urine).

Management

Treatment of invasive infections should be with intravenous benzyl penicillin. All strains are extremely sensitive to penicillin so that short courses of antibiotics are acceptable; treatment may be discontinued 48 hours after the child becomes apyrexial. Chloramphenicol should be combined with penicillin in children with meningitis until culture confirms meningococcal infection.

Children in whom meningococcal infection is suspected, especially in the presence of a petechial rash, should be given penicillin by their GP before transfer to hospital, particularly when the journey is a long one. Intravenous injection is preferred to intramuscular administration.

All household and day-care or school contacts should receive rifampicin, as should the index case, irrespective of whether meningococci can be isolated from the nasopharynx. Such prophylaxis should be given to contacts as soon as possible after a definite diagnosis has been made. Medical staff involved in mouth-to-mouth resuscitation should also be treated.

Vaccination should be considered when there is a cluster of cases occurring at the same time. Vaccines against groups A, C, Y, and W-135 are available (C on a named-patient basis), but only that to group A is effective under the age of two. Many recent cases have been caused by B serotypes for which there is no immunization available. A B vaccine is being evaluated at present.

Molluscum contagiosum

Organism

A poxvirus.

Epidemiology

A common infection which most individuals have at some time. Since lesions may be innocuous and then resolve, this mild infection is frequently missed.

Transmission

is by direct contact, the incubation period is from two to seven weeks and infectivity is low.

Natural history

The virus results in a characteristic pearly papule with an obvious central dimple. Size varies from 1 to 5 mm. These can occur anywhere in children, most commonly in small crops due to direct contact. They will always resolve eventually, usually within nine months.

Diagnosis

Diagnosis is clinical.

Management

'Anti-wart' solutions available from chemists are ineffective. More drastic local treatments are not justified since the lesions will resolve spontaneously. If they occur in the child's genital or peri-anal area the possibility of sexual abuse should be considered. However, lesions may have spread to those areas from a child's hands.

Mumps

Notifiable disease

Organism

The mumps virus.

Epidemiology

This is endemic and common in the UK. Infections occur throughout childhood but are unusual in the first year of life. By adulthood most individuals have been infected. Complications of mumps infection result in the admission of approximately 1400 people (all ages) to hospital in the UK each year. There is no evidence that infection during pregnancy results in congenital abnormality.

Transmission

is by airborne droplet spread.

Incubation period

is 16–20 days.

Infectivity

is high lasting from six days before to four days after swelling of the glands.

Natural history

The symptoms of mumps include headache, fever, and malaise followed by painful swelling of the parotid and/or submandibular salivary glands. The enlargement may be unilateral and assymetrical. Illness is subclinical in approximately 30 per cent of infections. Complications are relatively common and include meningo-encephalitis (sometimes as the presenting feature), pancreatitis, deafness (rare), and painful involvement of the testes and ovaries in adult sufferers.

Diagnosis

In its classical form, mumps is unmistakable. Other organisms may cause a parotitis or nearby lymph-node enlargement. Anti-body tests are available but seldom needed.

Management

This is symptomatic with analgesics where required. Only children with severe complications need to be admitted to hospital, where they should be isolated from immunosuppressed children, although even in this group the illness is rarely severe.

This will be a preventable disease once MMR immunization is introduced.

Nits *(Pediculosis capitis)*

Organism

Pediculus humanus capitis (head louse).

Epidemiology

This infestation is more common in areas of poverty, but nits are found amongst all social classes. Both nits (eggs) and lice are found in the hair.

Transmission

is by direct contact. The eggs take about nine days to hatch.

Infectivity

is high between household contacts and play-mates. The louse seems to be less common in Afro-Caribbean hair, it is thought because the different shape of the hair shaft makes nit attachment more difficult.

Natural history

After hatching the larva grows to maturity in nine days. It then feeds by sucking blood from the scalp and lays eggs (nits) which are cemented to the base of the hair shaft. The symptoms are an itchy scalp, though the child may not complain where infestation is light.

Diagnosis

The tenacious eggs stuck to the hair shaft are unmistakable; however the inexperienced observer may misidentify dandruff as nits, or vice versa.

Management

Two agents are active against head lice: malathion (Prioderm or Derbac) and carbaryl (Carylderm). Both are applied as lotions to the scalp and allowed to dry naturally (hair dryers will inactivate the drug). The hair should not be washed for 12 hours. The hair needs combing to remove nits and a repeat treatment in 10 days may be required as eggs can be resistant to treatment. The hair of close contacts should be examined and treated. Many areas operate a policy of rotating malathion and carbaryl treatment every few years to prevent drug resistance developing.

Children with nits or lice should not necessarily be excluded from school as older individuals are not very infectious to their peers until close contact resumes in adolescence. However, to ensure treatment it is often useful to have a local rule of exclusion until the first course is given.

Routine screening of school populations by nurses has not been shown to be of value. Their time is more usefully spent confirming diagnosis when suspected by teachers or parents, and then organizing treatment.

Pneumococcal infections

Organism

Streptococcus pneumoniae, a Gram-positive coccus. Also known as
the pneumococcus.

Epidemiology

This is the usual cause of lobar pneumonia and common cause of
acute pleural effusion in childhood. Many individuals are carriers of
the organism in the upper respiratory tract; disease occurs in
association with a viral upper-respiratory-tract infection or in the
presence of a particularly virulent strain. Certain groups of children
are at high risk of severe and sometimes fatal infection. These
include children with nephrotic syndrome, sickle-cell anaemia, or
after splenectomy. Patients with congenital or acquired immunodeficiency are also at risk.

Transmission

is from droplets of respiratory-tract secretions or recently soiled
handkerchiefs.

Incubation period

is 1–3 days.

Infectivity

is low in most cases and isolation is not required.

Natural history

Pneumococcal pneumonia is normally lobar. Infection in the right
upper lobe may be associated with meningism, and lower-lobe
infection with abdominal pain. *Streptococcus pneumoniae* is a

cause of meningitis (which may occur from the neonatal period into adulthood) and acute otitis media. Septicaemia may occur in the immunodepressed and in children with functional asplenia. Recurrent episodes of meningitis suggests chronic leakage of CSF.

Diagnosis

This is by identification of Gram-positive diplococci on Gram stain of secretions or following culture. Blood cultures may be helpful, and a polymorphonuclear leucocytosis is characteristic. Rapid diagnostic antigen-detection tests are available (latex-agglutination) but there is no evidence that they are any more sensitive than culture methods.

Treatment

Benzyl penicillin (150 mg/kg/day, 4-hourly) is the drug of choice for severe infections in childhood, with a minimum of 10 days for meningitis, and longer courses required in the presence of effusions or in the high-risk groups. Phenoxymethyl penicillin (penicillin V) is the drug of choice for lobar pneumonia in childhood. So close is the association with *S. pneumoniae* that treatment should be started before identification of the organism, although appropriate specimens should be collected for culture first (blood for culture and antigen detection, throat swab). Because of the poor absorption of oral penicillin, some clinicians prefer to give an initial dose of benzyl penicillin by intramuscular or intravenous injection. Where there is a clear history of penicillin allergy (rare in childhood) erythromycin can be given. Isolation is unnecessary.

Prevention

Children in the risk groups should be given anti-pneumococcal vaccine (Pneumovax) and prophylactic penicillin (see section on Special children, p. 256).

Poliomyelitis

Notifiable disease

Organism

Poliovirus, an enterovirus of three main types: 1, 2, and 3.

Epidemiology

A viral illness rare in the UK but endemic in many developing countries, especially the Indian subcontinent where annual incidence rates are estimated at 10–30 per 100 000 population. Because of the success of routine immunization, wild virus is rare in Britain and the majority of the few clinical cases now result from reversion of attenuated forms of the live vaccine, which can affect either the child being immunized or its unimmunized close contacts. From 1970 to 1984 only 70 definite cases, with two fatalities, were reported amongst residents of England and Wales.

Transmission

is by the faecal–oral route; food and water contamination is extremely rare and maintained swimming pools do not offer any risk.

Incubation period

is 7–14 days for paralytic cases.

Infectivity

via the faeces may be prolonged for six weeks or longer but is highest in the few days around the onset of symptoms.

Natural history

In children cases are often subclinical or simply show as a mild febrile illness. However, wild or reverted attenuated virus can invade the nervous system causing meningitis or selectively attacking the motor cells in the spinal cord causing paralysis which can be permanent or fatal. Adults are more at risk of such complications.

Management

There is no specific treatment for the paralytic form apart from bed rest in the acute phase. It is essential to ensure that all individuals in contact are themselves immunized.

Rabies

Organism

A rhabdovirus.

Epidemiology

This disease is endemic in the animal population in most developing countries and much of Europe. Only six cases were notified in England and Wales between 1977 and 1987; three of those were in children bitten by dogs in the Indian subcontinent.

Transmission

is by bite, or lick of broken skin, by a rabid animal.

Incubation period

is 2–8 weeks. The more severe the bite and the closer the distance between the site of the bite and the brain, the shorter the incubation period.

Natural history

The child will present with fever followed by a deteriorating neurological status including anxiety, confusion, convulsions and death. There will be a history of exposure to a rabid animal (usually lethal in the animal).

Diagnosis

Where possible, the suspect animal should be killed and brain samples tested for the virus. If the animal is still healthy two weeks after the bite/lick, there is no rabies risk. Specimens from the child (isolation of virus from saliva or CSF) rarely provide more than confirmation of a clinical diagnosis obvious by the deteriorating state.

Management

(See Travel abroad, p. 275.)

Respiratory syncytial virus (RSV) infection

(See bronchiolitis, p. 10)

Organism

This is an RNA, paramyxovirus.

Epidemiology

Infections are most severe in the first few months of life. Infants at particular risk of severe infection are preterm, or with congenital heart disease. Smoking by one or more parents appears to increase susceptibility to infection. Infection occurs in epidemics normally in winter and spring, at a time when the highest rates of the sudden infant death syndrome are recorded, suggesting a possible role of this virus in its aetiology.

Transmission

is from respiratory-tract secretions, and man is the only source of infection. It has been shown that the virus may remain viable for up to six hours in secretions outside the body.

Incubation period

is 5–8 days.

Infectivity

lasts about seven days from onset of symptoms.

Natural history

This is the most important cause of bronchiolitis during infancy.

In the preterm infant, signs may be non-specific and include lethargy and apnoea. In the term infant, signs are more localized to the respiratory system, with rapid breathing, intercostal recession and over-inflation of the upper chest. Auscultation with a stethoscope reveals crackles and wheezes. Complications include respiratory and cardiac failure.

Diagnosis

Nasopharyngeal aspirates can be sent to the laboratory early in the course of the infection for either culture or a rapid diagnostic procedure such as immunofluorescence, which has a higher sensitivity.

Management

Most infants with bronchiolitis can be managed at home. With more serious infection, hospital admission may be required for observation and tube feeding. Measurements of arterial gases may be required; hypoxia should be corrected with oxygen. A rising carbon dioxide level is a warning that intermittent positive-pressure ventilation may be necessary. Fluids should be restricted and electrolytes carefully monitored in severely ill infants. Diuretics should be used if heart failure develops. A newly developed anti-viral agent, ribavirin, has been shown to produce a marginal improvement in severely affected infants with congenital heart disease or bronchopulmonary dysplasia, and may be indicated in this group. This has to be administered as an aerosol and is extremely expensive (£800 for a three-day course). Infants should be isolated and careful handwashing employed to prevent spread to other hospitalized infants.

Prevention

Attempts at preparation of a vaccine have been unsuccessful.

Ringworm (Tinea)

Organism

Various fungal organisms of species *Microsporum* and *Trichophyton*.

Epidemiology

A widespread slow or chronic infection occurring in four clinical forms (see Natural history), some of which (scalp and body ringworm) may be acquired from animals.

Transmission

is by direct or indirect contact with infected lesions, including skin or hairs which have been shed. Hence it is possible to acquire scalp ringworm from shared pillows, and athlete's foot from shower floors. Body and scalp ringworm may be caught from dogs, cats, and other animals.

Incubation period

is variable, often prolonged.

Infectivity

lasts as long as lesions persist.

Natural history

Scalp ringworm (Tinea capitis)

This starts as a papule and spreads outwards, forming a scaly patch of temporary baldness. The hairs that remain are brittle. There may be progression to a general raised boggy mass (a kerion).

Body ringworm (Tinea corporis)

This is characterized by spreading ring-like lesions with a red, scaly periphery (sometimes with vesicles). As a lesion enlarges the centre often clears to leave normal skin.

Nail ringworm (Tinea unguium)

The nail(s) become discoloured, thick, and brittle. Some white material may accumulate under the nail which itself may eventually disintegrate.

Foot ringworm (Tinea pedis, athlete's foot)

Scaly itchy lesions develop between the toes (may also occur between fingers). This is more common in older children.

Diagnosis

Except in the easily diagnosed athlete's foot, a skin scraping should be collected. This is done by using a sharp blade to scrape a number of scales from the active edge of the lesion in scalp or body ringworm, or from under the nail. These should be collected onto black (or at least dark) paper and sent to the laboratory for microscopy and culture. Since the characteristic fungal hyphae are usually easily seen under the microscrope, diagnosis can be very rapidly done and reported by telephone.

Management

Scalp ringworm

Although topical treatment can be attempted in many cases this is unsuccessful and a systemic oral anti-fungal agent (griseofulvin) should be used for at least six weeks.

Body ringworm

As for scalp ringworm. Also give a topical anti-fungal preparation (clotrimazole) for two weeks, but impress on the family that the oral medicine is more important.

Nail ringworm

Oral medication (griseofulvin) is essential for up to six months to clear what can be a very persistent infection. Topical medication is ineffective.

Athlete's foot

Unless infection is very extensive, oral anti-fungals are not necessary. Give topical anti-fungal powder or cream (clotrimazole or econazole) and suggest that the feet are kept dry. When many cases of athlete's foot are being reported check whether standards of hygiene need to be improved in the local school or swimming pool.

Roseola infantum (exanthem subitum)

Organism
Probably human herpes virus 6 (HHV6).

Epidemiology
Occurs world-wide as a disease of infancy and early childhood.

Transmission
incubation period, and period of infectivity are all unknown, but unethical experimental studies were performed in the late 1940s in which serum from infected babies was inoculated into healthy infants who developed the illness in nine days.

Natural history
The child has a sudden onset fever with irritability. This lasts 3–5 days with the fever climbing to 40–41°C. The fever suddenly falls and a widespread maculo-papular rash appears (Fig. 2, p. 15).

Diagnosis
Diagnosis is clinical.

Management
Rule out more serious illnesses: see Child with a fever (p. 22–4) and Child with a rash (p. 13–21); otherwise symptomatic treatment.

Rubella (German measles)

(See Congenital infections: management during pregnancy and the neonatal period)

Organism
Rubella virus.

Epidemiology
Rubella infection in Britain is endemic and epidemics occur every few years (Fig. 5). Infection peaks in the late winter and early spring. In the epidemic years 1978–9 (seven years after the immunization programme was introduced) there were 131 cases of congenital rubella infection, approximately 10 per 100 000 live births—and since then there have been on average 33 cases per year. Eighty per cent of cases suffer defects, and pregnancies at particularly high risk are those of Asian mothers who arrived in this country in their teens and who were not reached by the school immunization programme. A large number of terminations of pregnancy (80 per annum on average in the past decade) are still performed following rubella infection during gestation.

Transmission
is from nasopharyngeal secretions or urine.

Incubation period
is 14–21 days.

Infectivity
persists from seven days before to seven days after development of the rash in postnatal rubella, while congenitally infected infants may continue to excrete virus for up to a year.

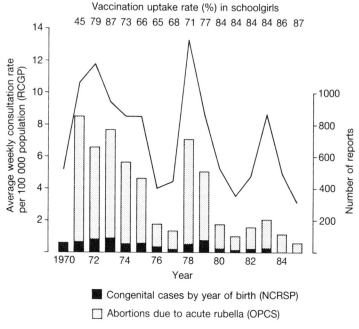

Fig. 5 Rubella, England and Wales 1970–75.

Natural history

Child and adult infection

Prodromal symptoms of infection include a sore throat, cough, and coryza, which may precede the rash by 1–5 days. The rubella rash appears first on the face and spreads to the rest of the body over the next 24 hours (see Fig. 2, p. 15). It is erythematous, and maculo-papular. The lesions on the trunk may coalesce to produce a red blush but those on the limbs remain discrete. The rash appears, spreads and disappears more quickly than that of measles. The rubella rash may be difficult to distinguish from scarlet fever, but in the latter the area around the mouth is spared (circumoral pallor) and the lesions are purple-red rather than pink-red in colour. Enlargement of the posterior auricular and occipital lymph nodes is a characteristic feature of the infection. Arthralgia may occur and encephalitis is a rare complication.

Congenital infection

Maternal infection up to the 18th week of gestation may result in the congenital rubella syndrome, (CRS) although lesions other than deafness are rare after 12 weeks. CRS is associated with intrauterine growth retardation; thrombocytopenic purpura; congenital heart disease, particularly patent ductus arteriosus; and pulmonary arterial or valvar stenosis. Sensorineural deafness is the most consistent abnormality and occurs in about 30 per cent of infected infants. Severe mental retardation associated with microcephaly and cerebral palsy may occur. Inadvertent immunization just before conception or during the first trimester of pregnancy has not resulted in CRS.

Diagnosis

The clinical diagnosis is difficult to make and may be confused with erythema infectiosum (see p. 55–6). Suspected rubella during pregnancy, or contact with an infected case, should be investigated using serological tests. Antibodies to the IgG subclass are measured at intervals of 10 days with a radial haemolysis test in acute and convalescent sera, and where there is a fourfold rise confirmation of infection should be made by a measurement of IgM. Many laboratories perform an IgM test initially when rubella infection is suspected during pregnancy. Infection in the neonate can be established either by viral culture of naso-pharyngeal secretions and urine or by serology.

Management

Treatment of rubella in the child or adult is entirely symptomatic. Equally, there is no therapy for congenital infection, but where this is known to have occurred before 18 weeks' gestation termination of pregnancy is recommended. Inadvertent immunization during pregnancy is not an indication for termination. When intra-uterine infection is identified, careful hearing tests, including auditory evoked potentials, should be performed during infancy so that, if required, hearing aids can be fitted at the earliest opportunity. Rubella infection will not recur in subsequent pregnancies.

Confirmed or **suspected** cases of CRS should be reported to one of the two central registries of the Congenital Rubella Surveillance Scheme as follows:

Thames, Wessex, South-western, Oxford, East Anglia, and Scotland

Dr Helen Holzel, Dept of Microbiology, Hospital for Sick Children, Great Ormond Street, London WC1N 3JH. Tel. 01–405 9200, Ext. 305.

West Midlands, Trent, Mersey, North-western, N. Yorkshire, and Wales

Professor R.W. Smithells, Dept of Paediatrics and Child Health, D Floor, Clarendon Wing, Leeds General Infirmary, Belmont Grove, Leeds LS2 9NS. Tel. 0532–432799, Ext. 3909/3900.

Immunization

(See also p. 200–3, 217–220.) Available for girls in secondary school. History of putative infection is not an excuse for omitting immunization, because a clinical diagnosis of rubella cannot be made with certainty. It is recommended that serology is checked before immunization in girls with arthritis, and vaccine should be avoided where there is active joint disease. Mumps/measles/rubella (MMR) immunization is to be introduced for pre-school children of both sexes in October 1988. Rubella infection is one of the few preventable causes of major handicap in childhood; health premises should display immunization posters and Asian women and other immigrants from less-developed countries should be targeted for education in this field. All health workers in contact with pregnant women should ensure that they are themselves immune to infection.

Scabies

Organism

A mite, *Sarcoptes scabiei.*

Epidemiology

Endemic in the UK, this infectious parasite is confined to humans, occurring in adults and children. It is much commoner where standards of hygiene are poor and bathing infrequent.

Transmission

is by direct contact or sharing of dirty clothes and bedlinen.

Incubation period

may be several weeks from first infestation to itching; with subsequent infestations the delay is much shorter.

Infectivity

is low but will persist until two courses of treatment have been completed. Mites and eggs in linen are inactivated by normal washing.

Natural history

The female mite burrows into the skin and lays eggs. The patient remains asymptomatic for several weeks until he or she becomes hypersensitive to the mite, whereupon intense itchiness develops which is especially troublesome at night. With subsequent infestations the itchiness comes on much earlier as the child's immunity is already primed. There are various signs of the infestation. The burrows of the female may be apparent; tiny wavy lines, sometimes with dark spots inside (the mite or her eggs). Most commonly these are in body folds: the finger webs, wrists, and elbows. When the hypersensitivity reaction has occurred papules, vesicles, or eczematous signs predominate but may be overlaid with the results of scratching. These lesions often occur away from the burrows e.g. on the abdomen and back.

Diagnosis

Essentially this is clinical. The diagnostic signs may be confused by scratching, inappropriate treatment (such as with steroids) and superinfection, and a trial of specific therapy may be useful. If a mite is seen, it can be collected in a skin scraping and sent for identification.

Management

Benzyl benzoate is the traditional treatment, with two courses given to all the members of the household. The lotion is applied all over (except for the head and neck), left for 24 hours (without bathing) and then repeated two days later. Benzyl benzoate is mildly irritant in itself and while this therapy kills the mite and eggs it does nothing for the hypersensitivity reaction and itchiness. A preferable treatment is crotamiton (Eurax) which when applied in a similar manner to benzoate both inactivates the mite and its eggs and relieves the itching. A further alternative is monosulfiram (Tetmosol). However, though less irritating than benzoate it is not as effective in relieving itching as crotamiton. It is also essential to ensure that all potentially infested clothes and bedding are thoroughly washed or the problem will simply recur. Children with scabies should not necessarily be excluded from school, though so as to ensure treatment it is sometimes useful to have a local rule of exclusion until the first course of lotion is given.

Staphylococcal infections

Organism

Gram-positive cocci which grow on agar in grape-like clusters. *Staphylococcus aureus* is coagulase positive and *S. epidermidis* is coagulase negative. There are many different strains, many relatively benign, some highly pathogenic.

Epidemiology

S. aureus is carried in the anterior nares of many individuals and *S. epidermidis* can be isolated from the skin of most people.

Transmission

is most commonly person to person via the hands or from the nose.

Incubation period

is 1–10 days for the scalded skin syndrome (a severe generalized skin infection, commonest in the new-born, when it is known as Ritter's disease), but infection frequently arises following prolonged colonization of the mucous membranes of mouth or nose.

Infectivity

is low.

Natural history

Most abscesses and wound infections are caused by *S. aureus*. The umbilicus of the new-born will become colonized by *S. aureus* quickly after birth and, unless the cord is kept clean, omphalitis and then septicaemia may develop. This organism is a cause of furuncles and paronychia in the new-born and, more seriously, of staphylococcal pneumonia, characterized by cavitating lesions and empyema (a collection of pus in the pleural cavity). *S. aureus* is the organism isolated most frequently from the sputum of infants and young children with cystic fibrosis, and is a common cause of osteomyelitis and septic arthritis. Certain toxin-producing strains of *S. aureus* cause food poisoning, scalded skin syndrome, and the toxic shock syndrome (now less common, but associated with tampon use). *S. epidermidis* may colonize indwelling catheters and prostheses and cause disease. Thus *S. epidermidis* may cause meningitis in a child with a ventriculo-peritoneal shunt or septicaemia in patients with central venous catheters.

Diagnosis

By Gram stain, culture, and the coagulase test.

Treatment

Most staphylococci produce penicillinase which inactivates conventional penicillin. Hence the anti-staphylococcal drug of first choice is flucloxacillin, a penicillinase-resistant penicillin. Cephalosporins are less effective against most staphylococci. Where the organism is resistant to the penicillinase-resistant penicillins, or there is a clear history of penicillin allergy, vancomycin can be used. Fusidic acid is recommended in combination with another anti-staphylococcal antibiotic in treatment of bone infection or other severe infection. Drainage of free pus should be performed and foreign bodies removed in the presence of infection.

Prevention

In the new-born: handwashing by all attendants is mandatory to prevent epidemics of staphylococcal infection and this will reduce the frequency of other infections. Care of the umbilical stump varies in different centres but antiseptics such as hexachlorophane and chlorhexidine, or topical antibiotics such as polymixin, bacitracin, and neomycin can be used. Epidemic disease in the new-born nursery is rare but infected infants should be isolated. There is no indication for the treatment of carriers of methicillin-resistant *S. aureus* (MRSA) unless they are long-stay patients or medical staff, in which case topical nasal antibiotics such as 'naseptin' should be used. Many infants and children with cystic fibrosis are treated with oral anti-staphylococcal agents on a long-term basis.

Streptococcal infections

(Excludes *S. pneumoniae*; see p. 103)
Scarlet fever is a notifiable disease

Organism

Streptococcus agalactiae or group B streptococcus. This is a Gram-positive coccus and is beta haemolytic. (Beta haemolytic describes the clear zone around colonies of bacteria on blood–agar plates.)

Epidemiology

This organism colonizes the genital tract of up to 15 per cent of pregnant women in the UK. Early onset of disease occurs in about one infant for every 100 women colonized, and is more common in the preterm infant.

Transmission

to the new-born occurs *in utero* or during delivery, or may occur from the hands of attendants.

Incubation period

is about three days.

Natural history

Features of **early onset** disease in the new-born include shock, apnoea, and pneumonia. It may be difficult to differentiate such infection from severe idiopathic respiratory distress syndrome. The infection is rapidly progressive. Meningitis is the commonest presentation of **late onset** disease although arthritis, osteomyelitis, and otitis media may occur.

Diagnosis

By Gram stain and culture or antigen detection.

Treatment

Until definite infection with this organism is identified, broad-spectrum treatment should be given. Benzyl penicillin alone is the treatment of choice for both early onset and late onset infection (100 000 u./kg per dose). Recent evidence suggests that ampicillin in large doses to a pregnant carrier mother (2 g, 4-hourly) may prevent infection in the new-born. There is no indication for the administration of penicillin to well infants found to be colonized after birth, as this treatment is rarely effective.

Organism

Streptococcus pyogenes or group A streptococcus (beta haemolytic). There are at least 75 strains. These are characterized by the 'M' protein in the cell wall.

Epidemiology

Transmission

may occur following inhalation of infected droplets from infected patients or asymptomatic carriers. Impetigo normally develops following direct skin contact. Many of the group A strains are capable of producing rheumatic fever, and glomerulonephritis is associated with a smaller number of strains.

Incubation Period

for pharyngitis is 3–5 days, but is longer for impetigo.

Infectivity

from tonsillar or skin colonization may be prolonged.

Natural history

The most common manifestation is tonsillitis or pharyngitis. Scarlet fever patients develop pharyngitis and a characteristic rash produced by an erythrogenic toxin. This rash develops during the first day of fever, is dark-red in colour and quickly becomes generalized. Lesions are punctate, the size of pinheads, and give the skin a sandpaper-like texture. There is a generalized erythema on the face and forehead, but the area around the mouth is spared (circumoral pallor). Fever peaks on the second day and in untreated infection persists for another 3–4 days. The tonsils are enlarged and covered with exudate. There are characteristic changes to the tongue: for 1–2 days the dorsum is covered in a white fur; the papillae then become red and thickened, protruding through the coat to produce the 'white strawberry tongue'. By the fourth or fifth day the white coat disappears leaving a 'red strawberry tongue'. Petechiae can be seen on the palate during the illness. *Streptococcus pyogenes* is a common cause of otitis media. Glomerulonephritis, but not rheumatic fever, may follow skin infections, whereas both conditions may develop after untreated pharyngitis. Septicaemia, endocarditis, and septic arthritis are rare complications of infection.

Diagnosis

Throat culture is a more reliable method of identification than the rapid antigen identification tests.

Treatment

A throat swab for bacterial culture should be taken from children with acute tonsillitis prior to treatment with antibiotics and it is usually preferable to await the results of culture (available in 24 hours) before starting treatment, particularly as viral tonsillitis caused by adenovirus and Epstein–Barr virus (EBV) cannot be distinguished on clinical grounds. A throat swab should also be taken from children with scarlet fever, although antibiotic treatment can be started once the diagnosis is made. Administration of penicillin for 10 days in the original studies was shown to reduce the risk of rheumatic fever and glomerulonephritis. Penicillin V is the drug of choice, but erythromycin is a satisfactory alternative where there is a definite history of penicillin allergy. There is no indication for the treatment of carriers. Mild impetigo may be treated with topical antibiotics.

Isolation

To prevent epidemics, children should not return to school for at least 24 hours after the start of antimicrobial therapy.

Tetanus

Notifiable disease

Organism

Clostridium tetani a spore-forming, anaerobic, Gram-positive bacillus.

Epidemiology

Neonatal tetanus is a relatively common cause of death in some less-developed countries because of unhygienic birth practices and inadequate care of the umbilical cord stump. In the UK almost all women of childbearing age are immune, so that anti-toxin antibodies are transmitted to the fetus by the trans-placental route, but this is not the case in many developing countries where tetanus immunization is not performed. Neonatal and childhood tetanus have almost disappeared in the UK with only two notified cases in the three years 1981–3.

Transmission

is by the direct transfer of spores of *C. tetani*, which can be found in soil, and the excreta of animals and humans.

Incubation period

is four days to three weeks.

Natural history

Following contamination of traumatized tissue, burns, or the umbilical stump, spores multiply in anaeobic conditions and produce tetanus toxin which causes powerful muscle contractions, extreme irritability, and death. Case fatality rates in neonates are high.

Diagnosis

This is on clinical grounds. Though infection is more possible in extensive wounds, the wound/site of entry may be trivial. Bacterial culture is positive only in a small proportion of cases.

Treatment

This includes tetanus immune globulin (500–3000 u.), benzyl penicillin for 10–14 days, surgical-wound debridement where indicated, and supportive medical management. Diazepam has proved very beneficial in treating neonatal tetanus. (See also immunization, p. 221.)

Threadworms

Organism

Enterobius vermicularis, a white worm about 2–12 mm long.

Epidemiology

Swallowed ova develop in the small intestine and then colonize the colon. Female worms migrate through the anal orifice, usually at night. Each deposits up to 10 000 ova in the perianal region. There is no secondary host.

Transmission

occurs when scratching begins and eggs accumulate under the finger nails with subsequent spread to other children, parents, and household objects.

Natural history

Infection produces intense perianal itch and irritation, especially at night. This may result in disturbed sleep and screaming episodes on waking.

Diagnosis

Distinctive thread-like worms may be observed in stools. Ova can be collected by pressing adhesive cellophane tape (Sellotape) against the perianal region using a wooden spatula and then looking for eggs microscopically or with a powerful hand magnifier. The best yield occurs in the early morning and parents can be shown how to apply Sellotape which is then brought to the doctor.

Treatment

Piperazine salts or mebendazole as a single dose given to all members of the family. Piperazine should be given on two occasions 14 days apart. Mebendazole should not be given to children under the age of two, and is taken once only. Attention should also be paid to personal hygiene, with a daily bath and hands washed and nails scrubbed before meals.

Thrush (candidiasis)

Organism

Candida albicans, a fungus.

Epidemiology

The normal skin flora includes *Candida* as well as bacteria. Infections are common during infancy, particularly in babies treated with antibiotics, and babies given dummies which become colonized with *Candida* sp.

Transmission

is by direct contact from the birth passages in the new-born infant, or from other sources of infection later. Most infections develop from organisms already present on the skin.

Natural history

Most commonly, this presents either as a white, cheesy deposit in the form of small plaques which may become contiguous on the tongue and inside the cheeks of young babies or as a perianal infection. If severe, the oral infection may interfere with feeding. Nappy rash may also worsen through superinfection. In immuno-deficient children, infection is a much more serious problem with widespread severe infection of the skin and mucous membranes with systemic involvement.

Diagnosis

In normal babies the diagnosis is clinical. Because it is a common skin commensal, there is no point in taking samples for culture. The mouth deposit may be confused with milk curds; however, the latter are easily removed with a clean finger while thrush itself requires gentle scraping with a tongue depressor and may leave a bleeding point when removed.

Management

Oral thrush usually responds to nystatin or miconazole and the removal of a dummy if one is being used. Infected nappy rash requires an ointment containing the same agents, perhaps in combination with 1 per cent hydrocortisone.

Treatment of the immunocompromised patient may require both topical therapy and intravenous antifungal agents.

Toxocariasis (visceral larva migrans)

Organism

A nematode; the two main species are *Toxocara canis* and *T. catis*.

Epidemiology

Toxocara canis is a primary infection of dogs which is increasingly being recognized as a hazard to young children (aged 1–4 years) particularly those with pica.

Transmission

occurs when ova from dog faeces are swallowed.

Infectivity

is low. The organism cannot be transmitted from person to person.

Natural history

Symptoms include allergic phenomena such as intermittent fever and asthma. The larvae develop in the small intestine of the child and migrate throughout the body causing allergic phenomena, wheezing, eosinophilia, and splenomegaly. Larvae do not normally mature in the human host. Dead larvae may give rise to endophthalmitis (an eye inflammation) or retinal granulomata and result in loss of vision.

Diagnosis

Eosinophilia and hypergammaglobulinaemia are characteristic. A diagnostic enzyme-linked immunosorbent assay (ELISA) which detects *Toxocara* sp. antibodies is available.

Management

This is with diethylcarbamizine citrate for three weeks. Surgery may be needed to remove granuloma(ta) from the retina.

Prevention

Public education about the danger to young children in allowing public parks to become dogs' lavatories (already the case in most areas). Children's sandpits should be covered to prevent contamination with faeces.

Toxoplasmosis

Organism

Toxoplasma gondii—a protozoan.

Epidemiology

This is a common infection and about half the population of Britain have antibody by middle age. Postnatal acquisition is commonest, but transplacental transmission also occurs in about 30–40 per cent of primary infections in pregnancy, resulting in fetal death or congenital infection.

The incidence of congenital toxoplasmosis (CT) in one Scottish study was 0.5 per 1000 births, but the size of the problem in Britain is unknown because 80–90 per cent of cases are asymptomatic at birth, and because even symptomatic cases, unless presenting as the classic triad (see below), are probably both misdiagnosed and underdiagnosed. However, approximately 200–300 cases of toxoplasma eye disease (all ages), almost all caused by congenital infection, are reported annually to the Communicable Disease Surveillance Centre. Postnatal acquisition in early childhood is probably relatively uncommon (about 10 per cent of 10-year-olds have antibody) in Britain.

Transmission

is poorly understood but is probably by two principal routes: consumption of undercooked meat containing the tissue cyst of *T. gondii*, and direct contact with soil contaminated with the oocyst stage of the organism's life cycle which is shed by domestic cats during acute infection. There is some evidence for transmission via unpasteurized milk (particularly from goats) and via water.

Incubation period

depends on the infecting dose and is probably about 10–14 days.

Period of infectivity

Infection is not transmitted from one individual to another.

Natural history

Postnatal infection

90 per cent of patients are asymptomatic and the remainder develop a glandular fever-like or non-specific febrile illness. Occasional severe systemic invasive infection is more likely in the immunocompromised patient but can occur in the immunocompetent. Complete recovery is usual, but tissue cysts and antibody persist for life. Reactivated cysts may lead to recurrent disease if the host becomes immunocompromised.

Congenital infection

80–90 per cent of infected infants are asymptomatic at birth, but almost all will develop chorioretinitis (can be after many years) and many will have varying degrees of neurodevelopmental retardation. If symptomatic at birth, the 'classic triad' of hydrocephalus, chorioretinitis, and intracranial calcification is virtually diagnostic but very rare; most often, non-specific signs such as prematurity, jaundice, hepatosplenomegaly, and thrombocytopaenia are seen.

Diagnosis

Postnatal infection

by serology—a specific IgM assay is available, or rising titre of IgG in paired sera.

Congenital infection

mainly by serology—cord or neonatal blood. The sensitivity of the IgM test depends on the assay method and even the best is not always reliable; it is therefore essential in suspected cases to measure IgG in serial samples at three- to six-monthly intervals in the first year of life, even if no IgM is detected. Levels usually remain high or increase following congenital infection.

Management

Postnatal infection

This is usually symptomatic only. If severe systemic disease occurs or if toxoplasmosis is diagnosed in pregnancy, specialist referral and advice from the Directors of Toxoplasma Reference Laboratories at PHLs in Tooting, Swansea, and Leeds (see p. 315), and the Dept of Microbiology, Raigmore Hospital, Inverness, for Scotland, is required.

Congenital infection

The effectiveness of specific treatment of toxoplasmosis diagnosed in infancy is unknown; children require specialist referral and advice. Treatment involves courses of pyrimethamine and sulphadiazine with folinic acid and of spiramycin (not licensed in the UK) throughout the first year of life. Long-term serological and clinical follow-up is essential.

Prevention

This is directed at preventing acquisition in pregnancy and can be summarized: 'Wash your hands thoroughly before eating or touching your face (particularly in the company of cats) and cook your meat thoroughly (brown right through).'

Tuberculosis (TB)

Notifiable disease

Organism

Mycobacterium tuberculosis. Also referred to as an acid fast bacillus
(AFB) (see Diagnosis). Atypical (non-tuberculous) mycobacterium
causes milder disease.

Epidemiology

Incidence and mortality are now low in the UK, having fallen as
living standards have risen. Estimates of incidence taken from a
survey of cases in 1983 in different racial groups were as follows:
white 2.6/100 000, Indian 34/100 000, Pakistani/ Bangladeshi 54/100
000. Second-generation immigrants are at lower risk and rates in
West Indian children are not demonstrably higher than in white
children. Certain groups of children are at high risk of infection:
those in close contact with active (especially open pulmonary) TB;
children recently coming from less-developed countries; children in
British Asian and African families.

Transmission

is by airborne spread from sputum of infected contacts with open
pulmonary TB. Unpasteurized milk may allow transmission from
infected cows.

Incubation period

from infection to primary lesion is 1–3 months.

Infectivity

is low. Usually this requires prolonged, close contact (e.g. sharing
living accommodation). Infection through brief contact is extremely

rare. Children are, on the whole, much less infectious than adults. When a case occurs in a school it is more important to look for the infecting adult, and the child should be isolated only if a sputum smear is positive. Tuberculosis affecting organs other than the lungs is not a risk to others. More commonly the problem arises as to how long to keep parents with 'open' TB away from their children. In this situation BCG (Bacillus Calmette–Guerin vaccine) should be given to the child and the parent(s) regarded as non-infectious following a few weeks of treatment, this being checked by smear testing of sputum. Where parent–child separation is undesirable, e.g. a mother with her new-born, treatment may be commenced in the asymptomatic baby (see p. 142).

Natural history

The organism almost always enters via the respiratory tract and primary infection occurs in the lung (primary focus, Ghon complex). Usually there is complete resolution or a small area of calcification following some localized inflammation (pneumonitis) and enlarged lymph nodes (hilar lymphadenopathy).

This process commonly goes undetected as the child seems well. Children may, however, become unwell if the infection proceeds, although mild disease can be undistinguishable from a simple respiratory infection with fever. Unless a tuberculous cause is suspected (e.g. known contact) the diagnosis may be missed. In a small number of children, there is direct spread to the lungs (bronchopneumonia), systemic spread to the lungs and other organs (miliary TB), or localization of infection following systemic spread to the meninges, bone, or kidneys. If infection is acquired by drinking infected (unpasteurized) milk abroad, cervical lymph node disease or gastrointestinal TB occurs. Malnourished children and those who have not had BCG are more likely to progress to severe disease.

Diagnosis

When tuberculosis is suspected, the child should be referred to a paediatrician who is likely to consult a chest physician or infectious disease specialist once the diagnosis has been made. Investigations should include a CXR and a tuberculin skin test: either a Heaf test (see p. 226–7) or a Mantoux test, in which 0.1 ml of 1 u. 1000 tuberculin, 100 u./ml is injected intradermally. The Mantoux test is positive when the diameter of the area of induration is more than 6 mm 48–72 h after the test has been performed. Weaker reactions may be due to prior BCG, infection with atypical (non-tuberculous) mycobacterium, or early disease.

A definitive diagnosis can be made by identification of acid fast bacilli, using the Ziehl–Nielsen stain; these may be seen on gastric washings, sputum, pleural or cerebrospinal fluid, urine, or other body fluids. These specimens should be cultured but the tubercle bacillus grows slowly and a positive result may not be obtained for up to six weeks. Further identification of infection may be made by histological examination; giant cells and tubercle bacilli may be seen in biopsy specimens from infected children.

Tuberculous meningitis is diagnosed following examination of cerebrospinal fluid (CSF). Most commonly there is a lymphocytosis, though early on neutrophils can predominate or the specimen may occasionally be cell-free; protein concentration is usually high and glucose low (under 50 per cent of value in blood taken simultaneously). If TB meningitis is suspected, the laboratory must be told so that the special stains and culture can be performed. The CSF should always be cultured so that the sensitivity of the organisms can be determined. It may sometimes be difficult to make the diagnosis from CSF examination and a tuberculin test should be performed immediately.

Management

This should be performed jointly by a paediatrician and chest physician or infectious disease specialist.

The new-born infant

There is rarely a need for separation of the mother with TB from her infant; breast feeding is not contraindicated during treatment with antituberculous drugs. The alternative forms of management in well babies are dependent on the disease status of the mother, as follows.

Mother with positive tuberculin test and no evidence of active disease

(assuming the mother has not been immunized previously): BCG can be given either at birth or within the first week of life.

Mother with positive tuberculin test and undergoing treatment for primary tuberculosis

Isoniazid should be given for six months to one year and isoniazid-resistant BCG administered after birth. The infant should be separated from the mother **only** while she is considered infectious (usually 2–4 weeks after the start of treatment).

Mother with haematogenous TB, such as miliary TB, TB meningitis

Following investigation of the infant to exclude congenital TB, give isoniazid for 6–12 months and isoniazid-resistant BCG after birth.

Infant with congenital TB

Treat with isoniazid and rifampicin for a minimum of nine months. **BCG should not be given to any baby delivered to an HIV-positive mother** because of the risk of 'BCG osis'. BCG does not produce immunity to TB in all infants and for this reason some physicians use chemotherapy alone in the new-born.

Later infancy and childhood

When a child is found to have a positive tuberculin skin test and there is no previous history of BCG immunization or evidence of active disease, isoniazid should be given for 12 months.

Children with pulmonary TB are best treated with a nine-month regimen; isoniazid and rifampicin are the drugs of choice. When it is thought that drug resistance is a possibility (and this is uncommon), a third drug should be added for the first two months of treatment: ethambutol, pyrazinamide, or streptomycin can be used. Ethambutol may cause an optic neuritis, which resolves if the drug is stopped in the early stages. Regular visual tests have to be performed, but interpretation may be difficult in the younger child so the drug should not be used in children under the age of six. Streptomycin causes vestibular and cochlear damage, the risk increasing with higher cumulative doses, so it should not be used for more than two months. Pyrazinamide may cause hepatitis; the preparation available in the UK is not licensed for use in children but is acceptable and has a place in the treatment of tuberculous meningitis (see below).

Miliary TB and tuberculous meningitis, as well as TB in other extra-pulmonary sites, should be treated with a minimum of three drugs: ethambutol, or pyrazinamide, or streptomycin given for the first two months should be combined with isoniazid and rifampicin, which should be given for a minimum of 18 months. Pyrazinamide reaches therapeutic concentrations in the cerebrospinal fluid and is used in both the UK and USA for children with tuberculous meningitis. There is no place for intra-thecal treatment in this condition.

Typhoid fever

Notifiable disease

Organism
Salmonella typhi, a bacterium.

Epidemiology
There are between 50 and 60 notifications of typhoid fever in children each year in England and Wales; most disease is acquired overseas, chiefly in the Indian subcontinent.

Transmission
is by contaminated food or water through the faecal–oral route.

Incubation period
depends on the size of the infecting dose. The usual range is 1–3 weeks.

Infectivity
Untreated cases may excrete the organism indefinitely after recovery, and asymptomatic carriers can be an important source of infection for long periods.

Natural history
The disease is usually mild in infants and more serious in older children and adults. Severe cases have sustained fever of insidious onset with malaise. Illness is associated with either diarrhoea or constipation and cough. Physical signs include hepatomegaly, splenomegaly, and rose-red spots on the trunk.

Diagnosis

This is primarily by blood cultures, but the organism can sometimes be cultured from stools or urine. Serological tests do not have a place in diagnosis.

Management

If this disease is suspected, rapid referral to a paediatrician is mandatory. Treatment will include intravenous fluids and chloramphenicol (see Gastroenteritis, p. 62). The Medical Officer of Environmental Health needs to be involved urgently for contact tracing.

Warts and verrucae

Organism

The human papilloma virus (HPV) or warts virus, of which there are a number of sub-types. Certain sub-types of HPV are associated with genital warts.

Epidemiology

Occurs world-wide in adults and children.

Transmission

is by direct contact, but with low infectivity. There is no good evidence that verrucae can be acquired from swimming-pool floors. The warts virus can be transmitted sexually.

Incubation period

has a large range from one month to two years.

Infectivity

may last as long as lesions persist.

Natural history

The appearance of warts is well known. It is less frequently appreciated that verrucae are warts occurring on the feet (plantar warts). The latter may be tender or associated with a 'pricking' sensation. Warts elsewhere are usually painless. The appearance varies with site: on the hands, face, and knees warts tend to be smooth and flat; in the genital and peri-anal regions they are larger, filiform, and fast-growing (condyloma acuminata); verrucae on the feet have the appearance of warts growing inwards.

Diagnosis

This is clinical. DNA analysis may be used to type a genital wart in cases of suspected sexual abuse.

Management

Commercially available medications are ineffective and the local treatments that do work (curettage, freezing, high concentration podophyllin) are painful and potentially hazardous outside special-ist hands. Most lesions resolve spontaneously and do not require investigation and treatment. Exceptions are genital warts, which may be acquired following sexual abuse. (Some genital sub-types of HPV may be associated with cervical carcinoma.) Children with genital warts should be referred to a paediatrician. Other exceptions include painful verrucae, hand warts interfering with writing, and facial warts causing distress to adolescents; children with these lesions should be referred to a dermatologist. There is no good reason to exclude children with verrucae from swimming or to force them to wear special socks.

Whooping cough (pertussis)

Notifiable disease

Organism

Bordetella pertussis, a Gram-negative bacterium.

Epidemiology

Whooping cough remains a common childhood disease in the UK. Epidemics occur at four year-intervals with peak incidence during the winter months. The last was in 1985–6; the next will be in 1989–90. When immunization rates were relatively high, epidemics were only moderate in size. However, following loss of public and professional confidence in the vaccine, in 1974 immunization coverage declined to 30 per cent and the scale of epidemics was greatly magnified (Fig. 6). Notified mortality from pertussis is relatively low (64 deaths from 1976 to 1985); however, these figures may be an under-estimate because it is possible the disease may go undiagnosed in some infant respiratory and 'cot deaths' where the presentation is without a characteristic cough and whoop.

Transmission

is by droplet spread or direct contact with discharge from the nose and mouth (including soiled handkerchiefs). Older children and adults may also have the disease in an unrecognized form and transmit it to young children.

Incubation period

is 7–10 days.

Infectivity

is highest in the catarrhal stage, but can be prolonged for up to a

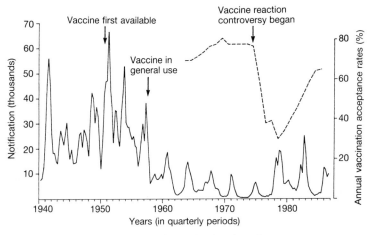

Fig. 6 Whooping cough, England and Wales 1940–86.

month after the start of the cough unless an appropriate antibiotic is given. When this is done, a child or adult becomes non-infectious in about five days (though the cough itself persists).

Natural history

Initially the child has a runny nose (catarrhal phase) followed in about two days by a cough which gradually becomes paroxysmal. During the bouts of coughing the baby or child may become red or blue/black in the face from hypoxia. One Asian word for the disease means 'the black cough'. When the bout stops, the child catches his or her breath, inspires in a rush, and causes the characteristic 'whoop'. Vomiting is common, and in young infants feeding may become impossible. Terminal apnoea is a significant risk in young babies following loss of consciousness with hypoxia. The cough gradually subsides, but bouts may persist for a number of months. A Chinese pictogram for pertussis can be interpreted as 'the illness of a hundred days'. Complications include pneumonia, encephalitis, convulsions, and cerebral damage.

Diagnosis

In a classical case this may be made on clinical signs as, once heard, the 'whoop' is rarely forgotten. However, it is important to confirm the diagnosis in all cases, particularly where the presentation is atypical, because other organisms (adenoviruses and *Bordetella parapertussis*) can produce similar illnesses. A diagnosis cannot be made using a throat swab. Instead a per-nasal swab (a swab on a four-inch flexible metal wand) should be inserted through the nose to take a sample from the back of the nasopharynx. This is unpleasant for the child and will often precipitate a bout of coughing. The swab is then placed in Stuart's medium and sent for culture or immunofluorescence. Because these swabs are positive in only about half the cases during the catarrhal stage of the illness, a negative result does not refute the clinical diagnosis. A substantial lymphocytosis is common in the early stages, but not diagnostic.

Management

Erythromycin given early in the catarrhal stage may shorten the illness. This antibiotic is recommended for all children with pertussis to render them non-infectious, which takes about five days.

The disease is hardest to manage in young babies where the paroxysms of coughing can be extremely frightening for the parents. To avoid vomiting, small, frequent feeds are advisable. Managing a baby at home can be both exhausting and stressful, and admission is often necessary for social reasons. When the child is having cyanotic attacks, admission is indicated for medical reasons because of the danger of terminal apnoea. In hospital the infant should be nursed in a cubicle until non-infectious. Tube feeding is often required. High levels of nurse staffing are needed because of the frequent attention these infants require when having coughing bouts. Microphone systems and apnoea alarms may be required to alert staff to an episode.

In the recovery phase the older child may be allowed to return to school. It will be necessary to explain to the teachers that despite its cough the child is not a risk to others. When a case or epidemic occurs strenuous efforts should be made to ensure that all contacts are up to date with their immunizations, if necessary using an accelerated schedule (see p. 313).

Yellow fever

Organism

An arborvirus.

Epidemiology

Yellow fever occurs in two endemic zones in Central Africa and northern South America with a natural reservoir in forest monkeys; however, cases occur in both urban and rural settings with a relatively high mortality. The disease is almost unheard of in the UK, but British travellers to endemic zones are at risk.

Transmission

is by mosquito, either between monkey and man or man to man.

Incubation period

is 3–6 days.

Natural history

A disease of varying severity which in severe forms manifests as sudden onset fever, malaise proceeding to jaundice, haemorrhagic symptoms, and death.

Diagnosis

This is by isolation of the virus or serological testing.

The collection of specimens for the diagnosis of infection

General principles

If in doubt whether to take a sample, what to take, or how to send it, the laboratory should be consulted first. As a rule, specimens should be collected only when results may affect management, or in the investigation of outbreaks of infection. The diagnostic tests for individual diseases are given in Table 11. In writing the request card remember that this is usually all the information that the laboratory has to go on. Therefore give details of:

the child's name and date of birth (not just his or her age);
the doctor's name, address, and telephone number;
the illness, its date of onset, and main clinical features;
treatment (particularly anti-microbials) and its duration;
relevant infectious disease contacts;
any recent foreign travel;
details (with dates) of previous samples.

Equipment

A clinic or practice will need the following:

swabs, including the per-nasal variety (see p. 159);
transport medium: Stuart's, chlamydial, and viral;
universal containers and 'dip slides' (if delay is anticipated);
faeces containers;
blood-taking equipment suitable for children ('butterflies', small-gauge hypodermic needles);
blood bottles suitable for small samples.

Table 11 Diagnostic tests for individual diseases

Disease	Specimen	Method of diagnosis
★ AIDS/HIV	Blood	Antibody test (Antigen test also done but expensive) Label 'High Risk' (red star). In acquired infection, antibodies may not be present for 3 months or more, although antigen can sometimes be detected earlier. Interpretation of results in children prior to 15 months is problematic because of antibody from the mother.
Chickenpox/ herpes zoster	Vesicle swab	Culture, serology, and electron microscopy of vesicle fluid available
△ Chlamydia	Neonates: eye swab or nasopharyngeal aspirate	Chlamydia transport-medium or special microscope slide.
	Older children: other swabs	Chlamydia transport-medium. Where sexual abuse suspected tissue culture must be performed (p.000)
★ △ Cholera	Stool/rectal swab	Diagnosis is by microscopy and culture; serology also available
Congenital cytomegalovirus	Urine Throat swab	Send promptly to lab.; serology inconclusive.
△ Diphtheria	Throat swab	**If suspected consult immediately.** If C. *diphtheriae* found, lab. will test whether a toxin-producing strain

Table 11 *continued*

Disease	Specimen	Method of diagnosis
Gastrointestinal infections:		
△* *Campylobacter*	Stool	Culture.
Cryptosporidium	Stool	Microscopy for cysts.
E. coli	Stool	Culture.
Giardia	Stool	Microscopy for cysts.
*in some cases (p. 000)		Need two or more specimens to exclude diagnosis; duodenal aspirate can be done in hospital.
Rotavirus	Stool	ELISA or electron microscopy.
△ *Salmonella*	Stool (not rectal swab)	Two specimens on separate days preferable for bacterial culture
△ *Shigella*	Stool	Bacterial culture.
Glandular fever or infectious mononucleosis	Blood	Full blood count and film will show lymphocytosis; serology using Bunnell or monospot test may not be positive for a month.
Haemophilus influenzae	Swab	Bacterial culture.
△ Hepatitis A	± serum	Clinical diagnosis sufficient in most cases; antibody tests are available but rarely justified.
△ Hepatitis B	Blood	Test for surface antigen.
△		Specimens must be marked 'High Risk' (red star).
★ Herpes simplex	—	Clinical diagnosis sufficient. Tissue culture is available but serology is not useful.

Table cont. on next page

Table 11 *continued*

Disease	Specimen	Method of diagnosis
Influenza	—	Clinical diagnosis sufficient. Viral culture of secretions collected on a nose or throat swab may occasionally be indicated.
★ △ Malaria	Blood	Examination of thick film or smear by an experienced person. This is an urgent investigation. Crucial to specify country of travel and anti-malarials taken.
△ Measles	Blood	Clinical diagnosis. Serology is available.
★ △ Meningococcal disease	Blood Cerebrospinal fluid (CSF)	Microscopy of CSF; bacterial culture; if suspected, for immediate referral (see p.000).
Molluscum contagiosum	—	Clinical diagnosis
△ Mumps	—	Viral isolation and serology available but normally unnecessary as clinical diagnosis straightforward.
★ △ Gonorrhoea	Neonates: eye swab Older children: swabs; put in medium to prevent drying.	See the child with sexually transmitted disease (p. 30).
Pneumococcus	Swab	Bacterial culture.
★ △ Polio	—	Urgent referral where suspected.

Table 11 *continued*

Disease	Specimen	Method of diagnosis
Respiratory syncytial virus	Nasopharyngeal aspirate	Immunofluorescence or viral culture.
Rubella	Blood (adult) Viral swab (new-born)	Serology in adult; culture in new-born
Staphylococcus aureus	Swab	Bacterial culture.
Streptococcal disease	Swab Serology	Laboratories will 'type' looking for group A haemolytic forms; antistreptolysin O titre useful in care of rheumatic fever and acute glomerulonephritis.
★ Tetanus	—	Urgent referral where suspected.
Thrush	—	Clinical diagnosis.
Tinea	Skin scrapings	Culture.
★ Tuberculosis △	Sputum Urine	Refer immediately when child is ill; if child is well perform Heaf test.
★ Typhoid △	Stool Blood culture	Culture for *S. typhi*.
Warts	—	Clinical diagnosis; DNA analysis where thought to result from sexual abuse.
Whooping cough	Per-nasal swab	Special swab on flexible wand inserted into the nasopharynx through the nose; put into Stuart's medium.
★ Yellow fever	—	Urgent referral if suspected.

★   Prior consultation of laboratory/paediatrician essential.
△   Contact the Medical Officer of Environmental Health who will initiate relevant contact-tracing and other preventive activities.
   Only routinely available tests are noted. Special tests are available for many of the diseases but will usually require consultation. Many of the infections listed are discussed in greater detail in the Diseases section.

COLLECTION—TRANSPORT—STORAGE

Blood

Most serological tests can be achieved with 2–5 ml, but it may be necessary to check with the laboratory the minimum amount required. An initial explanation that the patient is a child will often reduce the volume asked for. The sample can usually be stored at 4°C overnight. (Blood cultures are an exception, but these are rarely taken outside hospital.) Collection of blood from young children is not easy. Butterfly needles (green or blue) are useful because 'flashback' occurs once the needle enters the vein, and they tolerate greater movement of the child than ordinary needles before becoming dislodged. **Never collect blood from a vessel in the groin** and refer to an experienced children's doctor if sampling is difficult.

Skin scrapings

(Tinea) Collect for fungal hyphae by scraping with a blade from the edge of a lesion on to black paper (so that the white scrapings can be found), fold this carefully, put it in a universal container and send, requesting microscopy and culture.

Stool specimens

Where microscopy is required it is better to send fresh specimens. Optimal practice is to get samples for bacterial culture and viral identification to the laboratory the same day; if stored overnight this must be in a refrigerator at 4°C. On the request form it is particularly important to say whether a search for ova, cysts, and parasites is needed, and/or a culture, and whether the child has been anywhere abroad.

Swabs

Always put these into appropriate transport media. Apart from chlamydia and viruses (needing special media) all swabs can go in

Stuart's medium. Swabs from skin lesions need to be from an exudate or a damp area. This may mean lifting scabs or expressing pus/vesicular fluid. Throat swabs must be from the tonsils or any other area where an exudate or lesions are seen. Per-nasal swabs for detection of *Bordetella pertussis* require a special technique (see p. 150). Vaginal swabs should be collected from the vestibular fossa by gently drawing apart the labia minora. Rectal swabs need to be inserted just inside the anus. Specimens should, whenever possible, reach the lab within four hours. When overnight storage is unavoidable, keep them at 4°C; they must not be frozen.

Urine

In older children collect mid-stream samples using the same technique as for adults. In infants and younger children a clean catch specimen is best. This involves waiting with the partially naked child until he or she 'pees'. Then a sterile container is placed in the stream of urine. The technique demands infinite patience but it is far less susceptible to contamination than the stick-on urine bags. Drinks of orange and running taps help to speed up the process. Often it is most conveniently done in the clinic or ward by the parents. If a urine bag is used the perineum should be cleaned gently with water (not antiseptic) before this is applied. It is best to leave it exposed to view so that urine is removed immediately it is seen. Supra-pubic aspiration of urine with a needle and syringe is sometimes necessary but should be done in hospital.

Immunization

General introduction

Artificial immunity is achieved in two ways, active and passive. Active immunity is long lasting and is achieved with injected and oral vaccines. Passive immunity is short lived and comes from the injection of immunoglobulins. This section describes the principal vaccines and immunoglobulins available in the UK, their uses, and handling.

Vaccines are customarily divided into two groups: those that are live but attenuated and those that have been inactivated.

Live vaccines

BCG
Measles
Measles/mumps/rubella (MMR)
Mumps
Polio (oral form, OPV)
Rubella
Yellow fever

These are highly effective: by inducing a slight infection they give many years of protection, often from a single dose. Yet, apart occasionally from oral polio, the infection is not communicable to others.

Inactivated vaccines

Cholera
Diphtheria*
Hepatitis B
Influenza
Pertussis
Pneumococcus

Polio (injectable, IPV)
Rabies
Tetanus*
Typhoid

(*The vaccines for diphtheria and tetanus are preparations from the bacterial exotoxins rather than the bacteria organism itself. They are sometimes referred to as toxoid vaccines.) A single dose of inactivated vaccine tends to be less effective than a live preparation equivalent (notably so for typhoid and cholera) and multiple doses are usually needed to give long-term protection.

Increasingly vaccines employ sub-units of the pathogenic organism to promote a protective effect, and in the future we can anticipate entirely engineered synthetic vaccines. Despite this diversity, all vaccines work on the same principle: that by simulating response to a pathogen they induce active immunity. All the vaccines described below have been through a rigorous testing process before being licensed for use. However, there is no such thing as a perfect vaccine. Each has its own degree of effectiveness, indications, contraindications, and reactions, and immunizers must be aware of these or know where to find out details.

For each vaccine there is an immunization strategy. These fall into two broad types. Firstly, of protecting the susceptibles: this means providing immunity to individual children or adults at risk from the disease. This may be all individuals (e.g. for tetanus) or only a limited number (e.g. for pneumococcal disease). Secondly, that of reducing the circulation of disease-producing organisms. This works on a mass basis whereby if enough adults and children are vaccinated (high 'herd immunity'), and humans are the only host for a disease, then the organism may eventually die out, assuming there is no carrier state; or at least there will be little of the disease in circulation. Oral polio has worked in this way and the same could be achieved for measles and rubella.

CONTRAINDICATIONS

There are circumstances when vaccines must not be given, both general and specific.

General contraindications

Acute febrile illness

A temperature over 37.5°C (38°C rectally). If a child has an acute febrile illness, the immunization must not be given because, if the condition worsens diagnostic difficulties will arise as to whether the deterioration is due to the immunization or the illness. Since immunization is almost always an elective procedure, it is sensible to delay this until the child is well on the way to recovery.

Specific contraindications

The following contraindications and special considerations apply for all **live vaccines** (see list, p. 163).

Antibiotic sensitivity

All live vaccines contain minute traces of antibiotics necessary in their preparation, most commonly neomycin and polymixin. Extremely rarely, individuals have an anaphylactic reaction to a specific antibiotic and they should not receive a vaccine with the antibiotic concerned. However, most sensitivity to neomycin and polymixin is a mild contact-dermatitis or delayed hypersensitivity which are **not** contraindications.

Pregnancy

None of the vaccines in current use have been shown to cause fetal malformations. However, unless there are compelling reasons (e.g. an unprotected woman about to go to a yellow fever zone or endemic polio area) it seems wise to avoid immunization in the first four months of pregnancy. **It should be specifically noted that rubella immunization in early pregnancy is no longer a reason for advising termination** (see p. 117).

Giving multiple live vaccines

Two or more live vaccines may be given simultaneously (e.g. MMR). However, on theoretical grounds once one has been given

three weeks should elapse before the next live vaccine is administered (see also BCG, p. 229).

Immunodeficient children

A live vaccine may overwhelm a child who is seriously immunodepressed (see p. 258 for definition) and live vaccines should not be
given to such children. This does not apply to AIDS/HIV (see
p. 257).

Inactivated vaccines

(See p. 163–4 for list.) Attention must be paid to the contraindications for each vaccine, however the issues of antibiotic sensitivity,
pregnancy, and multiple vaccine administration are of less practical
significance than for live vaccines. Inactivated vaccines can be given
to all immunodeficient individuals.

Individual specific contraindications and children with problem histories

Individual vaccines carry a number of specific contraindications and
these are detailed below under each vaccine. When these apply, a
child must not be immunized. (An example is pertussis vaccine
where there has been a prior severe reaction.) There are also
circumstances (previously referred to as special considerations)
where immunization is perhaps thought to be associated with a
somewhat increased risk. These are referred to as children with
problem histories and detailed in the notes at the end of each
immunization section. An example would be immunizing a child
with a convulsive tendency with measles vaccine. Any additional
risk must always be weighed against the danger associated with
leaving the child unprotected. Each child needs individual assessment but, on balance, most children with problem histories should
be immunized. In the example given a British child with febrile
convulsions is 8–10 times more likely to suffer a further fit because of
measles disease than from the vaccine.

Adsorbed and plain killed vaccines

The three components of the Triple vaccine (diphtheria/tetanus/ pertussis) are available in plain form or adsorbed in an aluminium hydroxide suspension both in the individual (monovalent) and combined preparations. The one exception is monovalent pertussis which is available only in a plain form. Sometimes doctors use the plain form preparations where there have been local reactions to previous injections, as these seem to occur less frequently with the plain preparations. However, this is rarely an issue in children and, as a rule, the adsorbed should be used as it gives somewhat better protection.

Mythical contraindications

Both primary care and hospital practice are permeated with mythical reasons for children being denied protection. Unfortunately, many of these have been communicated to the public. The following conditions are **not** reasons for a child being denied protection through immunization.

The child (or any family member):
suffering from eczema, asthma, or hay fever;
receiving antibiotics;
receiving low-dose or topical steroids;
having a history of neonatal jaundice;
a baby being under a certain weight;
having a prior history of pertussis, measles, or rubella;
suffering from chestiness or snuffles;
suffering from 'underdevelopment';
having been born prematurely;
suffering from a stable neurological condition;
suffering from syndromes such as Down's or Turner's.

Likewise, there is no contraindication to immunization when a child's mother is pregnant or breastfeeding.

When a child is believed to have a contraindication to any immunization this must not be accepted on verbal basis alone. No indicated immunization must be denied to a child without careful verification by consulting this volume or the DHSS's *Immunization against infectious disease*. Where doubt remains specialist advice must be sought rather than omitting the immunization. Each Health District (Health Board in Scotland) has an individual designated as responsible for immunization and they will be able to deal with enquiries.

Vaccine handling

When vaccines are received from the pharmacy, chemist, or any other source they should be placed immediately in the main body of the refrigerator, not in the door section (where the temperature will rise on opening) or the freezing compartment. All vaccines must be protected from light. Maximum and minimum thermometers are necessary for vaccine fridges and these should be checked regularly.

TRANSPORT OF VACCINES AND USE IN SATELLITE CLINICS

Vaccines allowed to warm up will not work.

In many circumstances vaccines have to be transported by staff to peripheral centres before their use. When this happens they must be kept at their correct cold-storage temperature while in transit and at the peripheral centre. This is called a 'cold chain'.

Guidelines for maintaining a successful cold chain are:

1. Rigid cool boxes with well-fitting lids and two ice ('freezer') packs should be used for transport. Soft bags are not acceptable.

2. Excessive amounts of vaccine should not be taken out in cool boxes, and what is taken must be loaded into the cool box as close to the departure time as possible, so as to minimize the time out of the fridge.

3. Vaccines should be kept in the cool box with the ice packs throughout the session. The lid must be kept on the box as much as possible.

4. Unused vaccine should be returned to the main fridge as soon as practicable after the session is over.

5. Where repeated exposure of vaccines to higher temperatures has been unavoidable, they should be dated and used within two weeks.

Table 12 Required storage conditions for vaccines

Tetanus
Diphtheria
Dip./Tet.
Dip./Tet./pertussis
Hepatitis B
Pertussis
Adult diphtheria
Typhoid
	2–8°C
	Do not freeze
		Refrigerator, not
		  freezing
		  compartment

MMR Measles Rubella BCG	2–8°C **Do not freeze**	Dried MMR, measles, and rubella have a shelf-life of 2 yr at 2–8°C, but only 10 weeks at room temperature. BCG 1–2 yr at 2–8°C, but only one month at room temperature. All should be used within 8 h of reconstitution

Oral polio	2–6°C (Smith,
	  Kline, and
	  French)
	0–4°C (Wellcome)
		Refrigerator, not freezing
		compartment.
		Occasional exposure up
		to 25°C is permissible **but
		each exposure must not
		exceed 2 h**.
		(Oral polio vaccine may
		be frozen; bulk supplies
		are stored at −20°C)

Tuberculin PPD	2–8°C **Do not freeze**	Discard one hour after opening

Disposal

At the end of the session any prepared or opened vaccine must be
destroyed. The label needs to be defaced with a ballpoint pen and
the ampoules put into a 'burn bin'. Alternatively vaccines can be
returned to a pharmacy, in which case they should be transported in

a sealed bag within a pharmacy box. Burn bins should not be stored in satellite clinics but returned to the main centre.

Disposal of BCG vaccine and tuberculin PPD

Any remaining vaccine must be drawn into a syringe and placed in a burn bin for return to the health centre and incineration. Alternatively, it can be returned in a sealed box within a pharmacy box. Expired vaccines should also be placed in a burn bin or in a sealed bag in a locked box for return to the pharmacy.

Under no circumstances should vaccines, syringes, needles, or empty ampoules be disposed of in any way in the health centre/ clinic except by incineration in burn bins. They must not be put into ordinary waste bags and bins.

Accidental spillage of vaccine

Wash the contaminated surface with a suitable disinfectant, such as sodium hypochlorite 0.3–0.4 per cent (Chlorasol).

Preparing for immunization, medical prescriptions, nurse immunizing and parental consent

At the start of an immunization session, the vaccines, the equipment for vaccination, and the equipment and drugs for treatment of anaphylaxis must all be checked (see also p. 350).

Any child presenting for immunization has to be indiviually assessed by the nurse or doctor for: the indicated immunization; any contraindications; the child's fitness for immunization that day. If a nurse is immunizing and there is any doubt as to any of these points, or those on the checklist inside the back cover, she or he must consult a doctor rather than proceed with immunization or deny a child an indicated immunization.

Medical prescription

It is often considered that a written medical prescription is required for a child to commence a course of immunization, especially if immunization is then undertaken by nurses. Such a prescription can conveniently be given at a baby's six-week check.

Nurse immunizing

Nurses may immunize with or without the presence of a doctor as long as they are willing to undertake this professional responsibility and they have had adequate training in all aspects of immunization, including the indications and contra-indications of vaccines, the DHSS guidelines, and the recognition and treatment of anaphylaxis. For NHS-employed nurses there should be District Authority policies which the nurse should be aware of and adhere to. Health

Visitors should refer to the guidelines on vaccination and immunization issued by the Health Visitors' Association, 50 Southwark Street, London SE1 1UN.

Parental consent

This must be obtained for each and every immunization. Initial written consent, such as that often obtained by the health visitor at the birth visit, is a useful permanent record but is only an agreement for a child to enter a programme of immunization. Presentation of a child for immunization by the family may be seen as consent, though on each occasion parents should be given the relevant details of the immunization to be given and have any questions answered. Particular problems over consent may arise where the immunizers go to the child (e.g. in day nurseries or schools) and special care has to be taken that consent is given in these circumstances.

Parental counselling

Parents often hear incorrect ideas about the infectious diseases and immunization. The nurse or doctor needs to have the right answers to their questions. Some common queries are:

Q. *'There isn't much of these illnesses about these days.'*
A. Whooping cough is common, especially during epidemics, and substantial outbreaks occur every four years because immunization fell to below 40 per cent in children born in the 1970s. The same is true for measles because, nationally, uptake is well short of the 90 per cent needed for disease elimination. Rubella-damaged babies still occur, and it is only because British children are immunized against diphtheria, tetanus, and polio that these diseases hardly occur in this country.

Q. *'Only poor children get these illnesses.'*
A. The organisms are democratic and can affect any child.

Q. *'I'm going to keep my baby away from other children so he can't catch the germs.'*
   A. You can never fully protect your child by isolation. Adults can carry some of these illnesses without having any obvious signs of disease.

Q. *'They can treat all these illnesses these days.'*
   A. Babies still die from whooping cough and 10–20 older children succumb annually to measles, despite having the best hospital treatment. Children who recover can be seriously ill and can suffer from complications which have permanent effects.

Q. *'My child is a year old. Even if he gets one of these illnesses it won't affect him much.'*
   A. All the illnesses may be serious no matter what the child's age. British children who die from measles usually catch it beyond their early years and it is older unimmunized children who tend to spread

whooping cough to babies too young to be protected by immunization.

Q. *'I'm giving my child the homeopathic medicine against whooping cough.'*

A. The tests which have been done with this medicine suggest that it does not work. Indeed, it would be very surprising if it did as it is made from the sputum of someone with whooping cough which is then diluted many, many times.

NB: There are other 'folk' remedies for whooping cough which appear to be equally ineffective.

Q. *'These immunizations don't always work.'*

A. All the standard childhood immunizations give over 90 per cent protection to children receiving the full course. If a child catches the illness, he or she is likely to have only a mild form.

Q. *'Giving half the dose of immunization is safer, so let's try that first.'*

A. Anything less than a full dose may not give protection. A full dose is as safe as a half dose.

Q. *'Babies often get brain damage from the whooping cough injection.'*

A. The National Childhood Encephalopathy Study (the most extensive survey of reactions to whooping cough immunization) suggests that the risk of permanent damage from the whooping cough immunization (if it exists at all) is about once in every 310 000 injections. At this rate, a health visitor might expect one such child on her caseload once every 1500 years. The risk to an unimmunized child from the disease is currently about six times higher.

Giving vaccines

Equipment required

Appropriate syringe and needles, spoons;
vaccine to be administered;
toys;
'sharps' container (burn bin);
cotton-wool balls;
shock box (adrenaline, syringe, needles, and airway).

Reconstitution of vaccines and drawing-up

A new needle and syringe must be used for each injection.
Many live vaccines are freeze-dried and have to be reconstituted
with a diluent provided with the vaccine. It is essential that the
appropriate diluent is used. This should be added slowly to the
vaccine. Injection with excessive pressure will cause frothing which
is thought to make the vaccine less effective. The vaccine solution is
then checked to see that it is the correct colour (described in the
product insert). If it is not, it should be discarded and the vaccine
supplier (e.g. the community pharmacist) notified immediately.
Vials of preconstituted vaccines (e.g. DPT) should be shaken to
check there is no sediment (the 'shake' test). If there is, the batch of
ampoules should be returned to the pharmacy as it may have been
frozen at some point and rendered ineffective.

Skin preparation before injection

It is not necessary to swab the skin before injection. However, some
immunizers prefer to do so; they should use isopropyl alcohol
(Mediswabs, Sterets). For live vaccines (see p. 163 for list) the skin
should be allowed to dry (30 seconds is sufficient) before injection,

to avoid any possibility of the material used for swabbing the skin killing the vaccine. **Acetone should not be used for pre-injection swabbing: it is highly inflammable and thus a fire hazard.**

IMMUNIZATION CHECKLIST

Preparation

(These activities should preferably be performed out of sight of the parent and child.)

1. The immunizer washes his or her hands.

2. In the clinic a paper towel can be placed on the working surface. When in the patient's home a working surface can be prepared with a clean towel (paper or otherwise).

3. The vaccine expiry date and dosage must be checked.

4. The medical prescription and signature of the parent or guardian are checked (depending on local policy).

5. A 'shock box' for anaphylaxis must be available and its expiry date checked.

6. The syringe and needle are assembled firmly (otherwise the needle can blow off when injecting).

7. If the vaccine is in an ampoule this is broken using a cover (cloth) to protect the fingers. If it is in a rubber-topped vial, the top should be wiped first with a spirit swab. This is followed by waiting for 30 seconds to allow the spirit to evaporate before drawing up the vaccine.

8. Air is expelled carefully from the syringe.

Parents and child

1. The nurse or doctor must first check that the child and the records match and if the accompanying adult is not the parent

that they know the child sufficiently well to give a reliable history. The nurse or doctor must then explain the procedure to the child and parent/guardian, check that the injection to be given is indicated, and ask for any appropriate contraindications/special considerations, **especially prior reactions**.

2. The appropriate injection site is then selected in the anterior aspect of the thigh or deltoid muscle of the arm (see Fig. 7) and the child made comfortable (usually, for the younger child on an adult's lap, with one arm, the non-injection arm, around the adult's waist), removing clothing as necessary, and held firmly

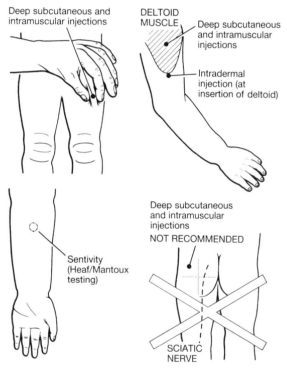

Fig. 7 Sites for vaccination.

so that if he or she flinches the movement will be minimal. Some parents choose not to be present at this point, and it is acceptable for another adult to hold and comfort the child during the actual injection.

Injection technique

Deep subcutaneous and intramuscular injections

The needle angle for intramuscular injection is 90 degrees to the skin, for subcutaneous injections 45 degrees. Once the needle has been introduced, the piston of the syringe is slightly withdrawn to make certain the needle is not in a blood vessel, then the vaccine is injected gently but steadily. When all has gone the needle is withdrawn. Many immunizers place dry cotton wool on the site and apply gentle pressure or rub for a few moments. A small leakage of vaccine, tissue fluid or blood from the vaccination site is common with sc or im injections and is not a cause for alarm. Cotton wool should be held on the site until the flow stops.

Intradermal injections

(BCG and Mantoux test.) (See Fig. 8.) A short (25 gauge—orange) needle is used. The skin is stretched and the needle inserted slowly with the bevel upwards for 2 mm into the skin almost parallel with the surface. The vaccine is injected cautiously. Resistance should be felt and a white blob begin to rise. **If both do not happen vaccination must stop and the needle be reinserted as it is probably too deep and there is a danger of giving a sub-cutaneous injection.**

After the injection the child is comforted (if necessary) and the parents told about mild reactions and how to manage them. The date when the next injection is due must be worked out with them and if they have a parent-held immunization record this is best filled in at this point.

Cleansing, replacement, and/or disposal

The needle must not be recapped as this is a potent source of needle-stick injuries. The needle, syringe, and ampoule (after recording the batch number) must all be placed in the burn bin as soon as possible. Empty vaccine packets, syringe packets, and needle caps can be put in an ordinary refuse bin.

Dosage

See Table 13.

Recording immunization

It is vital that immunizations be recorded in central and local records. The precise recording system may vary but the following

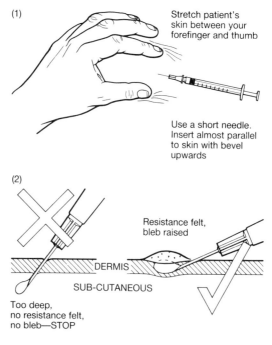

Fig. 8 Intradermal injection technique.

Table 13 Immunization doses (main vaccines only)

Vaccine	Route of administration	Usual dose	Recommended needle
Oral polio Triple Diphtheria/ tetanus MMR	Oral	3 drops	Nil
Measles Rubella Tetanus, diphtheria, or pertussis (monovalent) low dose diphtheria	Deep subcutaneous or intramuscular	0.5 ml	23G (blue)
BCG	Intradermal	0.1 ml (0.05 ml if under 2 years old)	25G (short orange)

For other immunizations, consult manufacturer's product inserts.

will be essential as a record of the immunization and that the correct procedure was followed:

Child identification (name, address, date of birth);
Date;
Type of immunization (DPT, Measles, etc.);
Place where immunization given (e.g. Radford Health Centre);
Batch number of vaccine (this may be kept in local records only);
Who gave the injection: a legible signature or printed name.

For the nurse and doctor's protection some District Authorities also suggest in their procedures that the immunizer make records along the lines of 'child fit for immunization—no contraindications'.

Immunization reactions

They are divided into three broad types: mild, severe, and anaphylactic. In addition, there are a few specific to particular immunizations and these are detailed in the descriptions of individual vaccines.

Mild reactions

Parents and older children must be warned to anticipate the commoner mild reactions: mild temperature, headache, general malaise, and local tenderness.

Severe reactions

These can occur after any immunization (or other drug). They are always rare but have been described more often after certain immunizations, most commonly pertussis and influenza. They can be local or general and are defined as:

Local: An extensive area of redness and swelling which becomes indurated (hard) and involves most of the front and side of the thigh, or a major part of the circumference of the upper arm.

General: A fever greater than 39.5°C occurring within 48 hours of injection or any one of the following occurring within 72 hours: anaphylaxis, bronchospasm, laryngeal oedema, generalized collapse, prolonged unresponsiveness, convulsions, or prolonged inconsolable screaming.

Anaphylactic reactions

These are even rarer than severe reactions but can occur after an injection of any drug or immunization, indeed they are much commoner with injected drugs. Though nursing and medical staff are unlikely to see a case of vaccine-induced anaphylaxis in their working life they must be prepared for the situation: first, by checking that adrenaline and the equipment needed to give it are available whenever immunization is taking place; secondly, by knowing how to identify anaphylaxis and to distinguish it from a faint; thirdly, by knowing what action to take should it occur.

The signs of an anaphylactic reaction are of sudden collapse with weak central pulses (femoral or carotid), profuse sweating, and loss of consciousness. Occasionally the onset is more gradual, perhaps with sudden swelling of the skin, wheezing, and difficulty in breathing before collapse. In the case of collapse, it is essential to check first that the child has not simply fainted (common in older vaccinees). This is done by checking the central pulses (carotid in the neck, femoral in the groin). The child or adult who has fainted will be pale but have a strong central pulse. Those worried about their ability to distinguish a faint from anaphylaxis should be reassured by the reports of the few who have seen the latter that they immediately knew what it was. If anaphylaxis is occurring (rapid or gradual onset), a doctor must be summoned **and** adrenaline injected subcutaneously or intramuscularly immediately. If oxygen is available, it should also be given. Nurses and doctors are strongly advised to familiarize themselves with the adrenaline dosages required for emergency therapy (see p. 350).

Reporting reactions

Severe and anaphylactic and other major reactions following immunization must be reported to the local Vaccination and Immunization administration giving:

Name of child and date of birth;
Address of the child;
GP of the child;
Nature of the vaccination;
Vaccine batch number;
The nurse/doctor who immunized;
Date of vaccination;

Where vaccination took place;
Details of the reaction.

A 'Yellow Card' needs to be filled in by a doctor for each severe reaction. This is then sent to the Committee on Safety of Medicines. Severe vaccination reactions brought to accident and emergency departments must also be reported, and the Yellow Card filled in by the doctor examining the child.

The reactions to the standard childhood immunizations are now described.

TRIPLE VACCINE:
DIPHTHERIA/TETANUS/PERTUSSIS, AND
MONOVALENT PERTUSSIS

Mild reactions

Up to 30 per cent of babies have a mild general reaction to immunization, or some 'local' swelling in the 48 hours after injection. Parents may find their baby has a slight temperature, general malaise and/or a red, sore, and swollen injection site. A mild analgesic such as paracetamol may be given. Sometimes a small lump is left after a local reaction; parents can be reassured that this will eventually disappear. These mild reactions are **not** a reason for withholding future pertussis injections.

Severe reactions

These occur only rarely. They can be local or general and are defined as:

Local: An extensive area of redness and swelling which becomes indurated (hard) and involves most of the front and side of the thigh, or a major part of the circumference of the upper arm.

General: A fever greater than 39.5°C occurring within 48 hours of injection or any one of the following occurring within 72 hours: anaphylaxis, bronchospasm, laryngeal oedema, generalized collapse, prolonged unresponsiveness, convulsions, or prolonged inconsolable screaming.

Handicapping reactions have been described following pertussis vaccine. This topic is discussed on p. 208.

A baby or child with a severe reaction must be seen by a doctor; the illness may be due to another cause unrelated to the immunization.

If a severe reaction occurs after a Triple or monovalent pertussis immunization, no more injections containing pertussis must be given. If it is not clear if a reaction is mild or severe, a doctor needs to make the final judgement. Details of the reaction need to be entered into the immunization notes. All other indicated injections can be given.

DIPHTHERIA/TETANUS, MONOVALENT DIPHTHERIA, AND TETANUS

Mild local reactions occur in young children following these vaccines but are less common than with pertussis. Reactions are more frequent and painful in older children, particularly with diphtheria vaccine (the reason for this is not clear) and after the tenth birthday a low-dose vaccine is given (see p. 190). Severe local and general reactions have been described, but are much rarer than with pertussis-containing vaccines in pre-school children.

MMR AND MEASLES

A mild general reaction 6–11 days after the injection occurs in a quarter to a third of children. There is occasionally a temperature and rash lasting up to 48 hours. The child is not infectious to other children. Very occasionally the fever may trigger a febrile convulsion. Children have also shown mild facial swelling 2 weeks after immunization. Severe reactions are extremely rare.

POLIO

Extremely rarely the vaccine may revert to its wild type and invade the nervous system (see p. 215).

RUBELLA

A few girls very occasionally experience some temporary joint pains as well as, or instead of, a mild general reaction (headache and feeling unwell). Severe reactions are extremely rare.

BCG

Mild reactions

There is normally a response at the vaccination site commencing within 2–6 weeks. Usually this is a small lump that enlarges and discharges some fluid to leave an ulcer. If this happens, a dry dressing should be applied but allowing air to the skin as this hastens healing. The discharge is not a source of tuberculosis to others. Children can go swimming though some authorities recommend an air-tight dressing while in the water. Some swelling and aching of the glands in the armpit often occurs temporarily. Deep ulcers are usually due to the BCG being given too deeply.

Severe reactions

Severe local reactions, suppurative adenitis, and osteomyelitis rarely occur following BCG and may be long delayed after the immunization. These must be brought to the attention of the doctor who may decide to consult an appropriate specialist with regard to therapy.

Individual immunizations

Not every vaccine available in the UK is covered in this section. For example, those used exclusively for adults, such as anthrax, will not be found here.

Those used only for travelling abroad are covered in the section on travel abroad.

Cholera immunization

Inactivated vaccine

Preparation

This is a heat-inactivated suspension of sub-types of *Vibrio cholerae* type 01. For availability and manufacturers, see p. 319.

Effectiveness

The vaccine is relatively ineffective in protecting individuals, and plays even less role in controlling infection at the community level. What limited protection is afforded lasts only 3–6 months.

Indications

The vaccine is scarcely ever indicated for any children. One or two countries still require certificated evidence of immunization (Niger and Qatar in 1988), though a single dose will suffice for this. Individuals are often given incorrect advice that they should have such protection.

Contraindications

Acute febrile illness or substantial chronic illness; age under one year; pregnancy; previous severe local or general reactions to a prior cholera injection.

How given

Im or deep sc injection. Children from 12 months to 4 yr are given a first dose of 0.1 ml, with subsequent doses of 0.3 ml; those aged five to nine, a first dose of 0.3 ml and subsequent doses of 0.5 ml; those aged over 10, a first dose of 0.5 ml and subsequent doses of 1.0 ml.

Reactions

Mild local reactions are common; general reactions very rare.

Diphtheria immunization

Inactivated vaccine

Immunization strategy

Protection of all susceptibles. The target is for 90 per cent of all children to have had three doses (within the Triple vaccine) by their second birthday.

Preparation

Diphtheria toxoid, preferably in its adsorbed form. This is normally given combined with tetanus and pertussis vaccines (Triple) but is also available with tetanus alone or on its own. A special low-dose monovalent preparation is available for adults and children beyond their tenth birthday. For availability and manufacturers, see p. 319.

Effectiveness

This is very high. The disease is confined to unimmunized individuals, although mild illness or asymptomatic infection may still occur.

Indications

All children

Every child should commence diphtheria immunization at three months and continue as per the national schedule (see back cover).

Unimmunized individuals

Older children (and adults) who have not been previously protected should receive the low dose diphtheria vaccine.

Contraindications

Acute febrile illness is a reason for deferring immunization for one week.

How given

Im or deep sc injection.

Reactions

These are extremely uncommon—usually local reddening with mild constitutional upset.

Notes

Booster doses for adults may be necessary as immunity from childhood immunization may not persist into adult life. If the person is going to a country where diphtheria is endemic, or there is a risk from exposure in an outbreak, it may be desirable to boost immunity by use of the low-dose vaccine.

Hepatitis B immunization

Inactivated vaccine

Immunization strategy

Prevention of perinatal transmission and protection of high risk susceptibles.

Preparations

Passive immunization

for immediate protection is afforded by hepatitis B immunoglobulin (HBIG) given as soon as possible after exposure and repeated one month later—now usually combined with hepatitis B vaccine (HBVac).

Active immunization

is given by an inactivated vaccine derived from the surface antigen of hepatitis B vaccine. Two types of vaccine are available, each containing 20 microgram/ml of HBsAg adsorbed on aluminium hydroxide adjuvant: (a) purified from human plasma; (b) produced by genetic engineering using a recombinant DNA technique. For availability and manufacturers, see p. 320.

Effectiveness

Combined passive and active immunizations are highly effective in preventing vertical transmission from mother to child. Active immunization is 90 per cent effective in providing protection to children, somewhat less for adults.

Indications and types of immunization given

Preventing perinatal transmission

—both active and passive immunization. Infants born to mothers known to be carriers of HBsAg (a component of the hepatitis B virus) which indicates the mother is potentially infectious to her infant and others. This is especially the case if she is also HBeAg positive (another viral component) and anti-HBe negative (that is, there are no antibodies to the HBeAg viral antigen). Such mothers are highly infectious. To identify them the following should be screened during pregnancy: ethnic groups other than Caucasian; all those where the history suggests increased risk of hepatitis B virus infection (principally intravenous drug abusers).

Protecting individuals exposed to infected blood (e.g. needle-stick injury)

—both active and passive immunization.

Protecting susceptibles

—active immunization.
Susceptible groups include the following:
Children and adults entering residential institutions for the mentally handicapped where there is known or likely to be a higher prevalence of hepatitis B infection.
Children and adults with chronic renal disease who are awaiting dialysis or transplantation. In immunosuppressed patients the immune response is likely to be poor so these patients should be protected as soon as they are considered for dialysis or transplant.
  Health-care staff: doctors, dentists, nurses, midwives, and others involved for more than six months in direct patient care of individuals suspected to be at higher risk of infection, especially staff who have direct contact with blood and body fluids through the use of, or contact with, needles and other sharp instruments. Immunization is particularly recommended for those working for longer than six months in units caring for known carriers of hepatitis B; laboratory workers and mortuary technicians; the staff of residential institu-

tions for the mentally handicapped (unless the risk is known to be low by serological testing); health workers (including students) involved in patient care in parts of the world with increased prevalence of hepatitis B (for practical purposes all less developed countries).

Some adult groups: active homosexuals and injecting drug abusers, if known to be non-immune.

Contraindications

1. Acute febrile illness is a reason for delaying active but not passive immunization.
2. There is no point in giving HBV to individuals who are already carriers (HBsAg positive).

How given

Active and passive immunization

—used following exposure to HBsAg-positive blood, e.g. where there is a risk of perinatal transmission or through needle-stick injury.

For new-born infants and children under 10 years, give HBVac 0.5 ml (10 microgram) im (anterolateral thigh or deltoid), repeated at one month and six months after exposure (intradermal use **not** recommended); plus HBIG 2.0 ml (200 mg) im (contralateral thigh or deltoid) as soon as possible after exposure. For perinatal infection HBIG should be given less than 12 hours after birth.

For children over 10 years (and adults) give HBVac 1.0 ml (20 microgram) im (deltoid is preferred site) repeated at one month and six months after exposure (alternatively, 0.1 ml (2 microgram) intradermally*) plus HBIG 5.0 ml (500 mg) im (contralateral arm or thigh; buttock may be used with special care in view of large volume) as soon as possible after exposure.

---

*Not yet recommended by the manufacturer but practised by some doctors.

Active immunization

Give HBVac 1.0 ml (20 microgram) im repeated after one month and six months to children under 10, and 0.5 ml (10 microgram) im repeated after one month and six months to children over 10. For rapid immunization, the third dose can be given two months after the initial dose with a booster at 12 months.

Reactions

Apart from a mild constitutional upset and some soreness and redness at the site of injection, no serious side-effects have been reported.

Notes

1. Intradermal injection

While the intradermal route for immunization is economically attractive for group vaccination as less vaccine will be used, the immune response may not be satisfactory should this more difficult injection technique not be carried out correctly. If this route is used, it would seem sensible to check the antibody response by serological testing.

2. Immunodeficient children

The HBV is safe for use in patients who are immunodeficient or immunosuppressed but the antibody response may be poor. An increased dose of the vaccine may be necessary to improve protection, and the serological response should be checked.

3. AIDS risk

No AIDS (or hepatitis) cases have been attributed to the vaccine prepared from human plasma and there is no risk of AIDS from the genetically engineered vaccine.

4. Post-immunization check

Some individuals do not respond to vaccination and, if risk of
exposure is high, it may be worthwhile checking immunity three
months after completing the immunization course to see whether
protective antibodies have appeared.

Influenza immunization

Inactivated vaccine

Immunization strategy

Protection of children with chronic respiratory and cardiac disease. Each year recommendations are made as to what strains should be included in the vaccines designed to provide some protection for the coming winter. The precise vaccine may, therefore, vary from year to year. Immunization is best carried out during the late summer or early autumn. The vaccines will not control epidemics and are recommended only for those at high risk.

Preparation

Vaccines are grown on chicken embryos and then inactivated. The precise composition varies from year to year. For availability and manufacturers, see p. 320.

Effectiveness

Current influenza vaccines produce reasonably good immunity, and are safe, being associated with only mild side effects.

Indications

Chronic lung and heart disease

Children with underlying chronic conditions involving the lungs (cystic fibrosis, severe asthma, and bronchopulmonary dysplasia) and heart (many forms of congenital heart disease). This is not done under the age of six months and is most commonly offered when the child enters school or day nursery where he will be in contact with a large number of other children.

Contraindications

1. Acute febrile illness is a reason for deferring immunization for one week.

2. Severe egg allergy. As the virus strains for vaccine production are grown in developing chick embryos severe egg allergy—angio-oedema, urticaria, acute respiratory distress, and collapse—is a contraindication. In assessing the risks and benefits of protection in a child reported to have such a condition, cautious skin testing may be useful before immunization.

3. Age under six months. No data are available on the use of influenza vaccine in infants under six months of age and they are not normally immunized.

How given

Primary immunization (6 months and older): two injections (0.5 ml) with an interval of 4–6 weeks. A booster injection should be given each year. When the recommended vaccine changes, only one injection is needed if prior immunizations have been received.

Reactions

Mild systemic and local reactions to the vaccine occur in up to 10 per cent of recipients, usually within the 6–48 hours after immunization. More severe reactions are uncommon.

Notes

1. Immunosuppressed children

Children who are no longer receiving chemotherapy are likely to have an adequate response with a high rate of seroconversion. If children are still receiving chemotherapy, the immune response is likely to be poor. The optimum time to protect children with malignant disease who must still continue their treatments is when they have been off chemotherapy for 3–4 weeks and when they have neutrophil and lymphocyte counts over 1000/mm^3.

2. Kawasaki disease or chronic arthritis

If these children require long-term aspirin therapy, influenza immunization should be considered because it is thought these children, if they acquire influenza, are at increased risk of developing Reye's syndrome.

Measles/mumps/rubella immunization (MMR)

Live vaccine

Immunization strategy

Protection of all susceptibles and national elimination of the measles, mumps, and rubella viruses. The target is for 90 per cent of children to be immunized by their second birthday, with similar or better levels among school entrants.

Following MMR's successful use in the United States and parts of Europe as a method of protecting susceptibles and minimizing the circulation of the three viruses, the vaccine is being introduced nationally in October 1988. It has been successfully tried out on a mass scale in three Health Districts (two in England, one in Scotland). The successful introduction of MMR is crucial for the control of measles and rubella. Individual districts and general practitioners have achieved the target of 90 per cent, but nationally measles immunization has only just reached 70 per cent. Hence, the disease has remained endemic with continuing child morbidity and mortality (see p. 91). The policy of selective female immunization against rubella has had higher uptake but has now reached the limits of its effectiveness, and an intolerable number of terminations for exposure to rubella are still having to be performed (see p. 115). Any further reduction in the number of rubella-damaged fetuses requires the reinforcement afforded by vaccination of children of both sexes in their second year of life, which with high uptake will reduce virus circulation. Also, mumps is a continuing source of substantial child and adult morbidity (see p. 99).

To be successful this new strategy will require high immunization uptake, beyond that presently achieved for measles.

Since the peak ages for catching all three diseases involve the pre-school and early school years, it will be essential to immunize as many children as possible in these age groups, otherwise virus elimination may take many years. This kind of coverage will be achieved by initially immunizing with MMR both at the normal age for measles (roughly 15 months) and at the same time as the pre-school booster (age 4–5 years). The vaccine will also be generally available for any children over a year (and adults) where requested. Children (and adults) who have already had measles, mumps, or rubella disease and children who have already been immunized with measles (or rubella) vaccine can all be immunized with MMR. There is no particular risk associated with 'double immunization'. As elimination of the virus will take time the policy of immunizing secondary schoolgirls and all sero-negative women must also continue in the immediate future.

Preparation

The freeze-dried vaccine contains three attenuated live viruses: the Schwartz strain of measles, the Urabe AM/9 strain for mumps, and the RA 27/3 strain of rubella. The measles and rubella components are currently in use in Britain in their monovalent forms, and the mumps vaccine has been licensed for some years.

Effectiveness

All individual components give long-lasting individual protection following a single immunization. (For measles and rubella this has been shown to last at least 20 years.) Effectiveness seems equally high when the vaccines are given together. With sustained herd immunity of over 95 per cent the United States has now minimized the circulation of virus to the point where all three infections are rare diseases.

Indications

Children aged 1–2 years

MMR will be given to children of both sexes in the second year of life (that is, at the time measles is offered now).

Children aged 4–5 years (pre-school booster)

MMR will be offered to children of both sexes at the time of their pre-school booster. This will entail two separate injections, MMR and diphtheria/tetanus (and polio drops). Where parents are reluctant for two injections to be given MMR should take preference and the diphtheria/tetanus be given later.

Children between two and four years, older children and adults

These will be given MMR when parents request.

Contraindications

1. Acute febrile illness is a reason for deferring immunization for one week.

2. Children with immunodeficient conditions must not receive MMR (see p. 258 for definition, and note this does not apply to HIV children, see p. 257).

3. A history of extreme sensitivity to neomycin or kanamycin is a contraindication because the vaccine contains traces of these antibiotics (see p. 165).

4. A history of anaphylaxis following exposure to chicken or egg products is a contraindication (but not the commoner forms of egg allergy: rash, diarrhoea). This is because the measles component is prepared on chicken fibroblasts and the mumps on eggs.

5. Pregnancy. Though no cases of fetal abnormalities have been reported as due to any of the vaccine strains, it is recommended not to immunize in pregnancy. If immunization happens inadvertently, it is not an indication for termination of the pregnancy.

How given

A single sc or im injection.

Reactions

Reactions are very similar to those following the present measles vaccination with a mild fever, malaise, and/or rash occurring in a quarter to a third of children, commonly in the period 6–11 days after injection, and lasting about 48 hours. The rash, if it occurs, follows a day or so after the fever and looks like that of rubella. The family should be warned to anticipate these reactions and told about temperature management (see Note 1 below). It should also be explained to them that the child with such a reaction is non-infectious. Children have also occasionally shown mild facial swelling 2–3 weeks after immunization, presumably due to the mumps component.

Notes

1. Child with a personal or close (first-degree relatives) family history of convulsions

These children must be immunized as they are at high risk of a convulsion when they catch measles, particularly if their history is of febrile convulsions. There is a much smaller risk (one-eighth to one-tenth) that a febrile reaction due to the immunization could also trigger a convulsion. Parents of such a child must be advised on temperature management when immunization takes place. If a temperature develops, various strategies can be employed depending on the severity of the convulsive tendency. Where risk is small, a combination of oral paracetamol, removing excess clothes, and keeping the room cool is usually effective.

The previous practice of administering immunoglobulin simultaneously with the injection must now be discontinued as this may limit the effectiveness of the mumps and rubella components of the vaccine.

2. Parent education

Since the MMR vaccine is new to families, there will be particular advantages in giving parents leaflets explaining its rationale and its associated mild reactions.

3. Exposure to measles—a measles outbreak

If a child is thought to have been exposed to measles and has not previously been immunized, then an injection of MMR given within 72 hours of exposure will lessen the impact of the disease.

Measles immunization

Preparation

A monovalent live attenuated virus. For availability and manufacturers, see p. 318.

This vaccine should now only be used where parents refuse MMR but still wish their child to have protection against measles. Contraindications are as specified for MMR (p. 200).

Mumps immunization

Live vaccine

Preparation

A monovalent live attenuated virus. For availability and manufacturers, see p. 321.

This vaccine has few indications for its use in isolation. Where parents specifically wish their child to be protected against mumps they should be strongly advised to use MMR vaccine.

Pertussis immunization

Inactivated vaccine

Immunization strategy

Protection of individuals and limitation of epidemics by high herd immunity. Target is for 90 per cent of all children to have had three doses (within the Triple vaccine) by their second birthday.

Preparation

A suspension of killed *B. pertussis* organisms, either combined with dipththeria and tetanus (Triple vaccine) or as a monovalent vaccine. For availability and manufacturers, see p. 321.

Effectiveness

Highly effective in protecting individuals from disease. One dose gives approximately 30 per cent protection; two, 60 per cent; three, 90 per cent. Disease is milder in those few who are infected after immunization.

Indications

All children

Every child should commence pertussis immunization at three months and continue as per the national schedule (see back cover) or by an accelerated schedule during epidemics (see p. 313).

Unimmunized individuals

Older children who have not been previously protected against pertussis should receive pertussis vaccine (either monovalent or combined, as appropriate) especially where younger children are at risk. An accelerated schedule should be used (p. 313).

Contraindications

1. Acute febrile illness is a reason for deferring immunization for one week.

2. A severe local or general reaction to a prior immunization including pertussis. Definitions:

Local: An extensive area of redness and swelling which becomes indurated and involves most of the front and side surface of the thigh or a major part of the circumference of the upper arm.

General: Any of: temperature over 39.5°C within 48 hours, anaphylaxis, bronchospasm, laryngeal oedema, generalized collapse, prolonged unresponsiveness, convulsions, or prolonged inconsolable screaming occurring within 72 hours of immunization.

How given

By im or deep sc injection.

Reactions

Mild reactions (irritability, local tenderness, and pyrexia) are common: 5–30 per cent depending on criteria. These are commoner with the second and third dose; however, it does not necessarily follow that a child who has had a mild reaction to one dose will react to following injections. A small, firm nodule frequently develops at the injection site. Parents can be reassured that this will either resolve or become impalpable as the arm grows. Severe reactions are uncommon but are considered more likely to re-occur. A connection between pertussis immunization and handicapping reactions (brain damage) was previously suggested, though with a very low frequency (one case per 310 000 injections, a rate equivalent to once every 1500 GP or health-visitor working years). **Recent reviews have** suggested there is no evidence for this link, certainly none for any causative association. It seems that in the well-reported cases where pertussis vaccine was thought to have caused damage, vaccination has happened to coincide with the sudden onset of brain disease. Parents concerned about the vaccine need this to be explained and to be reminded that complications after whooping cough are, in contrast, relatively common.

Notes

1. Children with problem histories

(1)   Children with a documented history of cerebral damage in the neonatal period;

(2)   children with a personal history of convulsions;

(3)   children whose parents or siblings have a history of idiopathic epilepsy.

Though the chances of reactions may be higher in immunizing these children, they should still be protected as benefits outweigh the risks. Parents of children in categories (2) and (3) should be instructed in methods of temperature control (paracetamol, stripping) to use if their child develops a fever so as to prevent this leading to a febrile convulsion.

Where the nurse or doctor is unsure as to whether to give pertussis or not they should rapidly seek specialist advice (preferably by phone) rather than deny the child protection.

2. Mythical contraindications

These are legion for pertussis (see p. 167).

3. Cerebral irritation and a history of convulsions

are no longer considered contraindications.

4. Stable neurological conditions

Children with stable handicaps (e.g. cerebral palsy or spina bifida) may be immunized.

5. Prior illness

Viruses can mimic pertussis. A child reported to have had pertussis should only be denied protection if diagnosis was confirmed by detection or isolation of *B. pertussis* (see p. 150).

6. Neurodegenerative conditions

It would seem wise not to immunize children with such conditions against pertussis. Note: children covered by Notes 4 and 6 will all be known to paediatricians and there will be value in discussing individual cases.

7. Oral homeopathic vaccine

This is prepared from the sputum of a pertussis sufferer. Having had multiple dilutions it probably does no harm but the evidence from the single published trial is that there is no protective effect.

Pneumococcal immunization

Inactivated vaccine

Immunization strategy

Given to individuals with conditions making them susceptible to severe pneumococcal infections. In normal adults and children the spleen makes a substantial contribution to protection against pneumococci. Children with absent or ineffective spleens are therefore susceptible.

Preparation

A capsular polysaccharide (cell-wall) extract of 23 sub-types of *Streptococcus pneumoniae*.

Effectiveness

The vaccine is relatively successful in preventing severe pneumococcal infections (pneumonia, meningitis, bacteraemia) in susceptible children beyond their second birthday. Antibody levels remain high for at least five years. It is ineffective under two years and no protection is afforded against commoner conditions where pneumococcus is sometimes implicated (recurrent otitis media).

Indications

Children with absent or deficient spleens

Children beyond their second birthday (and adults) with any condition involving lack of the spleen or loss of splenic function: sickle-cell disease (not trait), nephrotic syndrome, some immunodeficiency states, post splenectomy.

Contraindications

Acute febrile illness is a reason for deferring immunization for one week.

How given

A single dose by im or deep sc injection. No booster is recommended. When splenectomy is planned, vaccination should take place at least two weeks beforehand.

Reactions

About half of vaccinees report mild local symptoms. One per cent have fever, myalgia, or more severe local reactions. Anaphylactic-like reactions are extremely rare (estimated one per 200 000 doses).

Notes

1. Specialist consultation

Any child who might benefit from protection is likely to be known to a paediatrician, who should be consulted prior to immunization.

2. Children under two years

If at risk, these will need antibiotic prophylaxis until their second birthday and then vaccination. Whether to then continue antibiotics is a specialist decision.

Polio (OPV) immunization

Live oral vaccine

Immunization strategy

Protection of all individuals and minimizing wild (pathogenic) virus circulation in the community by high herd-immunity. Target is for 90 per cent of all children to have had three doses by their second birthday.

Preparation

Live attenuated vaccine combining the three strains of polio virus. For availability and manufacturers, see p. 327.

Effectiveness

Immunization gives protection both in the gut and systemically. The former reduces symptomless excretion and reduces circulation of wild virus. The three doses protect 95 per cent of individuals against the three strains of virus.

Indications

All children

Every child should commence polio immunization at three months as per the national schedule (see back cover).

Unimmunized individuals

All older unimmunized children and adults should use a catch-up schedule. This is most conveniently done by the general practitioner.

Previously immunized children and adults
travelling to endemic areas who have not had a booster in the
preceding 10 years should be given one before travelling.

Contraindications

1. Acute febrile illness is a reason for deferring immunization for
    one week.

2. Immunodeficiency (see p. 258 for definition) in a child, their
    siblings, or parents are contraindications and IPV is given
    instead because of the concern that the child or deficient family
    member would be at risk of infection from a live vaccine.

3. A child suffering from **acute diarrhoea** should have immuniza-
    tion delayed. However, vaccination should proceed if there is
    merely chronic loose stools (toddler diarrhoea).

4. Extreme antibiotic sensitivity. OPV contains traces of neomy-
    cin, streptomycin, and penicillin (though less than is sometimes
    found in doorstep milk). In the very rare circumstance of
    extreme hypersensitivity (anaphylactic) to these antibiotics a
    child should not receive OPV.

5. Pregnancy. There is no evidence of OPV ever having caused
    fetal damage. It is, however, advised not to be given to a
    pregnant woman in the first four months of pregnancy (though
    her children may be immunized) unless there is a compelling
    reason (e.g. an unprotected woman travelling to an endemic
    country).

How given

The vaccine is given orally, with three drops constituting a dose. It is
customary in schoolchildren to put the drops on sugar lumps. When
this is done care must be taken that large numbers of lumps are not
prepared in advance as some may be left in the warm for so long that
the vaccine is inactivated.

Reactions

Very occasionally (approximately once every 1–5 million doses) OPV will revert to its wild form in the vaccinee and cause polio disease in the child or a close contact.

Notes

1. Breast feeding

This does not interfere with vaccination.

2. Immunizing parents

It is impractical to immunize adults in child health clinics (Where is the immunization record kept?) and unprotected adults should be given the vaccine by their general practitioner.

3. Combining with inactivated polio vaccine (IPV)

Children from other countries and some adults will have had IPV. For purposes of completing courses and boosters IPV and OPV can be seen as interchangeable, and an adult who had IPV as a child and needs a booster can have a single dose of OPV.

Polio (IPV) immunization

Preparation

An inactivated combination of the three polio virus strains. For availability and manufacturers see p. 321.

Inactivated polio vaccine (IPV) is used in the UK only for immunodeficient individuals (see p. 258 for definition). It is also recommended for family contacts of such children. Other countries use it more extensively amongst healthy children. It is safe and gives good individual protection, though it may be less successful in preventing wild virus circulation. Like OPV it combines the three virus strains. It is given by im or sc injection as per the OPV schedule, but with only febrile illness, pregnancy, and extreme antibiotic hypersensitivity as contraindications. It is essentially interchangeable with OPV so that someone commencing a course with one vaccine may complete it with the other.

Rubella immunization

Immunization strategy

The protection of all susceptibles. The UK is presently adopting the MMR vaccine and so reinforcing current rubella immunization strategy with disease elimination. However, the schoolgirl immunization programme, routine blood-testing of adult women, and postnatal immunization of seronegative women will need to continue for a least 10 years from the general introduction of MMR, perhaps for longer.

Preparation

This is a live attenuated freeze-dried vaccine grown on human diploid cells. For availability and manufacturers, see p. 322.

Effectiveness

A single dose is considered to give protection for at least 20 years. Even though antibody levels decline over this period, there seems to be no fall in protection. A few women do not sero-convert (see Note 4 below).

Indications

All girls between their tenth and fourteenth birthdays

These children are usually immunized at school or in the GP surgery. A prior history of rubella disease is not a contraindication.

Seronegative women of child-bearing age

It is essential that all women in this age-group be tested for rubella antibodies.

Seronegative male and female hospital staff

This is to protect susceptible pregnant women in antenatal clinics. All health-service staff should therefore be screened for their immunological status.

Contraindications

1. Acute febrile illness is a reason for deferring immunization for one week.

2. Immunodeficient children and adults (see p. 258 for definition) must not be immunized.

3. Pregnancy is a contraindication. Some previous vaccines (now out of use in the UK) were considered teratogenic (producing malformations). However, their use has been discontinued and no malformations have been reported with the diploid vaccines in cases of immunization of susceptible pregnant women. Hence, although pregnancy remains a contraindication (at least a month should elapse between immunization and pregnancy), termination of pregnancy is **not** indicated when immunization inadvertently occurs.

4. Extreme antibiotic sensitivity to neomycin or polymixin is a contraindication (see p. 165).

How given

A single im or deep sc injection.

Reactions

Mild joint pains are common, occurring in up to 20 per cent of adults receiving vaccines but only 3 per cent of children. They commence any time from 3 to 25 days after injection (most commonly 8–14 days) and usually last 2–4 days. Mild general reactions are also common, with fever, sore throat, lymphadenopathy, and rashes. These are mild infections and are therefore delayed in onset. Mild transient neuropathies ('pins and needles') have also been reported, but more severe reactions are extremely rare.

Notes

1. Prior history of rubella

Diagnosis of rubella is often problematic and such a history is never a justification for withholding immunization for children. In a woman beyond her sixteenth birthday, policy is to check her rubella serology unless it seems likely that she will not return later. In that case immunization should be given without serology.

2. Children with joint conditions

Mild joint pain is a common reaction following rubella immunization, and exacerbation of childhood arthritis has been reported. Hence, it is worthwhile testing the rubella serology of any girl with such a condition prior to immunization (blood tests are usually being done anyway) as she may have achieved natural immunity. However, if the girl is non-immune she should be immunized.

3. Co-ordination of school and GP immunization

Secondary schoolgirls may be immunized in either setting. However, whenever a girl reports to one agency that she has been or will be immunized by the other this must be verified, so that evasion of immunization may be detected.

4. Negative serology despite prior immunization

Routine blood tests may fail to detect low antibody levels which still are protective for the fetus. Equally, however, the woman may still be unprotected. If there is a verifiable history of immunization, the problem needs to be explained to the woman and the case discussed with a specialist.

5. Postnatal immunization

Some seronegative women are detected in pregnancy by antenatal screening. They will need immunization after delivery. This can be done in the postnatal ward or at a postnatal check, unless a transfusion has been given in which case immunization should be delayed for three months. If anti-D (rhesus) immunoglobulin is also needed, the two can be given simultaneously at different sites.

6. Information for women

All women who are tested should be informed of their results in writing.

7. Immigrant women

Few less-developed countries offer rubella immunization, and women from these countries have been shown to be more often unprotected than their UK-born counterparts. This group therefore requires special attention, particularly because of their high fertility.

Tetanus immunization

Inactivated vaccine

Immunization strategy

Protection of all susceptibles. Target is for 90 per cent of all children to have had three doses (within the Triple vaccine) by their second birthday.

Preparation

A cell-free suspension of the inactivated toxin of tetanus, produced either on its own, combined with diphtheria and pertussis (DTP or Triple Vaccine), or with diphtheria alone. For availability and manufacturers, see p. 322.

Indications

All children

Every child should commence tetanus immunization at three months and continue as per the national schedule (see back cover).

Unimmunized individuals

Unimmunized older children and adults should receive protection using a catch-up schedule.

Following injury

See p. 254 in Practical immunization: questions and answers for a detailed discussion.

Contraindications

Acute febrile illness is a reason for delaying routine vaccination but vaccine should be given immediately if the indication is an injury.

How given

By im or deep sc injection.

Effectiveness

This is very high. Disease is now confined to the unimmunized. Immunity of pregnant mothers is transferred to the fetus and prevents neonatal tetanus. The adsorbed form is marginally more effective in conferring immunity than the plain preparation.

Reactions

Mild local reactions are common, especially in older children and adults. These can arise soon after injection or up to 10 days later. They may persist for a few days and require an analgesic, such as paracetamol. If the injection has been superficial, a nodule may be felt. This will eventually resolve. General reactions are uncommon and anaphylactic responses exceedingly rare.

Notes

1. Excessive number of doses

Since hypersensitivity reactions can occur, individuals should not receive large numbers of doses. Unless there is high risk of exposure, an adult need not be immunized at less than 10-yearly intervals.

2. Severe local reaction

This suggests good immunity and probably no further doses are needed for at least 10 years. If another dose is indicated the plain form should be used as it is less reactogenic. Some practitioners will first try skin testing with a dilute dose, though the usefulness of this is not certain.

Tuberculosis (BCG) immunization

Live vaccine

Immunization strategy

Protection of all susceptibles. Target is for 95 per cent of secondary schoolchildren to be tuberculin positive or given BCG. With declining disease incidence the broad mass of school-children are at decreasing risk; however, present policy is to continue routine school immunization. Incidence is also declining amongst Asian and African families but remains at a higher level than for the rest of the population. If routine immunization ceases, a programme will still be needed in every Health District for these groups.

Preparation

BCG (Bacillus Calmette–Guerin) in a freeze-dried preparation form. BCG is an attenuated mycobacterium (the family of bacteria causing tuberculosis). For availability, see p. 319.

Effectiveness

BCG is moderately effective. In adolescents, 70 per cent protection is given for 15 years. The degree of protection afforded by BCG given in the neonatal period is less certain, though it is thought to prevent TB spreading through the blood-stream and, in particular, to protect against TB meningitis.

Indications

High-risk neonates

This is done without prior sensitivity testing for all new-born infants (see HIV-positive children, p. 257) in contact with infectious cases of respiratory TB, or in families of ethnic Asian or African origin (not West Indian), or countries where TB is more prevalent (for practical purposes all less-developed countries). **In all other circumstances the child must be shown to be tuberculin negative before giving BCG.**

Some children acquire BCG immunity naturally. They do not need BCG and if they receive it can suffer a severe local reaction. This can be tested by seeing if the child's skin is sensitive to tuberculin, an inactive derivative of the TB organism. Groups to be tested and if tuberculin (Heaf/Mantoux) negative given BCG: all schoolchildren between the ages of 10 and 13 years (inclusive); close contacts of cases of infectious acute respiratory TB; health-service staff; students, including those in teacher-training.

Contraindications

1. Acute febrile illness is a reason for deferring immunization for one week.

2. Tuberculin-positive individuals.

3. Immunodeficiency (see p. 258), including symptomatic or asymptomatic HIV infection—this includes new-born and young babies of HIV mothers where the diagnosis cannot be made with certainty.

4. Generalized severe septic skin conditions.

5. Pregnancy. No cases of malformation have been reported. Where immunization inadvertently occurs, this is **not** a reason for advising termination of pregancy.

How given—sensitivity testing

Uses PPD (purified protein derivative). This is used in routine immunization but also for diagnosis and contact tracing. For the latter two, interpretation is difficult and requires specialist consultation.

Mantoux testing

(Suitable for individual patients.) Use 1 : 1000 dilution (100 u/ml). PPD given as an intradermal injection (see p. 186 and Fig. 8). Inject 0.1 ml.
Use only one needle and syringe per patient.

Heaf multiple puncture test

(Suitable for mass testing.) This uses a spring-loading 'gun' with six short needles set at 1 mm until a child reaches their second birthday, 2 mm thereafter. The PPD dilution (100 000 u/ml) is more concentrated than for the Mantoux test and is specially supplied in vials sufficient for about 50 tests. A variety of applicators may be used: a sterile platinum-wire loop, a sterile glass-rod, or a syringe and needle. With one of these a very small amount of PPD is put on the forearm (see Fig. 7 for site, p. 178). The applicator itself should not touch the skin. If it does, then re-sterilization (loop or rod) or changing (needle) is needed. The PPD is smoothed on the skin using the loaded 'gun' end-plate. The end-plate is held firmly at 90° on the skin and the 'gun' then fired. The needles of the 'gun' must be kept sharp and the 'gun' apparatus sterilized between each person by dipping its end-plate and needles in spirit and then passing these through a flame so that the spirit on the apparatus catches light and heat sterilization takes place. The gun should not be kept in the flame and it must be allowed to cool before the next child! This will take about 30 seconds. The gun must not become contaminated in this time. If necessary, it can be protected in a sterile tube. (Note: some Health Districts now use disposable heads for guns, removing any need for flaming.)

Interpreting the Mantoux

Read between 72 and 96 hours. A positive result is an **indurated** (hard) area of 6 mm or more diameter.

Interpreting the Heaf

Read between 72 hours and 10 days. Positive reactions are those of Grade 2 and above (see Fig. 9). A borderline (5 mm) Mantoux is equivalent to a Heaf Grade 2–3. In routine testing prior to immunization, a negative test indicates a need for BCG. A borderline result (Heaf Grade 2) means an individual is probably already immune. Those above Grade 2 require referral to a specialist to check that active disease is not present.

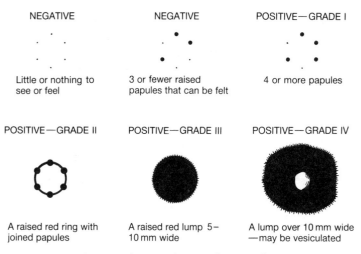

NEGATIVE

Little or nothing to see or feel

NEGATIVE

3 or fewer raised papules that can be felt

POSITIVE—GRADE I

4 or more papules

POSITIVE—GRADE II

A raised red ring with joined papules

POSITIVE—GRADE III

A raised red lump 5– 10 mm wide

POSITIVE—GRADE IV

A lump over 10 mm wide —may be vesiculated

Fig. 9 Guide to reading Heaf test results.

How given—BCG

Vaccine is reconstituted with supplied diluent and 0.05 ml (under 3 months) or 0.1 ml (all older individuals) given by intradermal injection (see p. 180 and Fig. 8) on the arm (customarily the left, see

Fig. 7, p. 178). **A separate needle and syringe must be used for each individual and jet-injectors are not to be used.**

Reactions

In most babies and children (and adults) there is a local reaction at the BCG site starting from 2–6 weeks after immunization. This begins as papules which can later discharge. No treatment is needed but parents may wish to use a dry, non-occlusive dressing. The child can still be bathed and go swimming (when a waterproof 'elastoplast' should be put on temporarily). This reaction is a local BCG infection and eventually heals leaving a small scar. More severe reactions do occur. They include prolonged deep ulceration, lymphadenitis, and osteomyelitis. **Their most common cause is faulty technique resulting in a subcutaneous rather than an intradermal injection.** Where these occur specialist advice must be sought.

Notes

1. Testing immunity after BCG

Immunity is not usually tested after immunization. A normal local reaction (see above) can be taken as indicator of success. High-risk individuals, e.g. health-service staff and children immunized at birth, may require sensitivity testing.

2. Skin disease

Individuals with skin disease so severe as to contraindicate BCG are extremely rare. With conditions such as eczema or psoriasis, PPD and BCG should be injected into disease-free skin.

3. Which arm?

It is customary to use the left arm (rather than the non-preferred) so that the eventual scar can be identified later.

4. Combining with other immunizations

As BCG is a live vaccine three weeks should elapse between it and any other live immunizations. In addition, immunization into the same arm should be avoided for three months as sometimes this results in painful axillary (arm-pit) lymph nodes.

Typhoid immunization

Immunization strategy

Protection of susceptibles.

Preparation

A monovalent vaccine of killed *Salmonella typhi*. For availability and manufacturers, see p. 324.

Effectiveness

This vaccine gives only moderate time-limited protection, lasting one year after a single dose, three years after two doses.

Indications

As the disease tends to be mild in children, and the protection afforded is only moderate, there is little justification for use of this vaccine in children. Good hygiene is much more important as a method of protection.

Contraindications

1. Acute febrile illness or chronic illness;

2. age under one year;

3. pregnancy.

How given

As im or deep sc injection: for children from one to nine years, each dose is 0.25 ml; for adults, 0.5 ml. The intradermal route is not used for the first injection, though it can be on subsequent occasions when the dose is 0.1 ml for all.

Reactions

Mild to moderate local or general reactions are common in adults, less so in children. General reactions are common. Where these are troublesome but immunization is considered necessary, the intradermal route is more likely to avoid discomfort.

Yellow fever immunization

Live vaccine

Immunization strategy

Protection of susceptibles.

Preparation

A freeze-dried preparation of live attenuated virus grown on chick embryos. This is only administered in designated yellow-fever vaccination centres and by a few general practitioners. A full list of centres is in the DHSS Memorandum *Immunization against infectious disease*.

Effectiveness

This is high, with immunity from a single dose lasting at least 10 years.

Indications

All children over nine months (and adults) travelling to or stopping in an endemic country. See the DHSS leaflet (Further reading, no. 13) for a current list of countries who require a certificate.

Contraindications

1. Acute febrile illness is a reason for deferring immunization for one week;

2. age under nine months;

3. immunodepression (see p. 258 for definition);

4. extreme hypersensitivity to neomycin or polymyxin, egg or chicken protein.

Reactions

Mild local or general reactions are relatively common, more severe reactions rare. Encephalitis has occurred in young infants, which is the reason for age under nine months being a contraindication.

Immunoglobulins given to children

Immunoglobulins give immediate but short-lived (passive) immunity. The preparations used in the UK are predominantly from human sources. Concern has been expressed that they could be contaminated by HIV (human immunodeficiency virus) and so cause AIDS. The preparation process of these products, however, is such as to kill this (and all other) viruses.

All immunoglobulins are given by deep im injection. Where volumes are large and the child is slim the buttock may be used (but with care to avoid the area of the sciatic nerve, see Fig. 7, p. 178).

Normal immunoglobulin

This is indicated in prevention of hepatitis A for non-immune travellers to highly endemic areas of the world (see p. 274). For protection of travellers the dosage for a period of travel under three months is 125 mg for a child under 10 years and 250 mg for anyone over 10. For a period of travel of 3–5 months the dosage is correspondingly doubled.

Note: Ideally, such immunoglobulins should not be given within four weeks of the live vaccines polio, MMR, measles, and rubella, or the toxoids diphtheria and tetanus.

Normal immunoglobulin is occasionally given to children with profound immunodeficiency. Such children will be under the care of a specialist who will decide on such therapy.

SPECIFIC DISEASES AND IMMUNOGLOBULINS

Chickenpox

ZIG (anti-varicella/zoster immunoglobulin). This is indicated for: immunodepressed children (see p. 258) in contact with chickenpox or zoster (shingles); babies born six days or less after onset of maternal chickenpox; babies whose mothers develop chickenpox in the week after delivery; babies in the first month of age who are in contact with chickenpox or shingles and whose mothers have no history of chickenpox.

Measles

Normal immunoglobulin given to immunodepressed children (see p. 258) exposed to measles. The dosage is 250 mg for babies under 12 months; 500 mg for those aged 1–2 years; and 750 mg for those over two years. A preparation of concentrated human measles immunoglobulin is available in Scotland.

Mumps

No specific immunoglobulin is now given or available. Immunodepressed children (see p. 258) may be considered for normal immunoglobulin if exposed to mumps.

Hepatitis A

See normal immunoglobulin, above.

Hepatitis B

Immunoglobulin is indicated along with hepatitis B vaccination (see p. 193) for infants of high-risk carrier mothers (those HBeAg positive or both HBeAg and anti-HBe negative). It is also given to infants whose mothers suffered acute hepatitis B in the last trimester of pregnancy or early in the postnatal period. The dosage is a single injection of 100 iu given as intramuscular injection. The appropriate immunoglobulin is available from the Hepatitis Epidemiology Unit, Central PHLS (see p. 315) and may be repeated at monthly intervals if active immunization is delayed.

Rabies

See p. 275–7.

Rubella in pregnant contacts

Normal immunoglobulin is sometimes given to pregnant contacts of rubella but is of little proven efficacy. The dosage is 750 mg.

Tetanus

Tetanus specific human immunoglobulin (Humotet) is occasionally given to severely injured under-immunized children. The dosage is 250 iu (1 ml).

Practical Immunization:
Questions and Answers

Practical immunization: questions and answers

How to use this section

This section is designed to give individual answers to many of the simple problems encountered in day-to-day immunization practice. Nurses and doctors engaged in such work will find it useful to read through the section completely. However, each question is written so that it can be read individually and hence there is a degree of repetition in the text. Readers should be aware that though in most cases the correct answer to a specific problem is to offer all indicated immunizations, there are many parents, doctors, and nurses who have been misinformed and will believe the contrary. The information and opinions they have been given are examples of **immunization myths**, for a full list of which see p. 167.

Counselling parents

In many of the situations described, parents will be seeking guidance from professionals. Families require different degrees of counselling and the nurse advising parents will need to judge which parents are particularly confused by the myths or have other concerns which are best discussed with a well-informed doctor. General practitioners and community children's doctors may occasionally have to consult community or hospital paediatricians or other specialists. Whenever possible this should be by telephone so as not to delay immunization. **It is never justifiable to deny a child protection out of ignorance.** The practice of giving diphtheria/tetanus alone and 'we'll check about pertussis' must not be undertaken. Experience is that children do not catch up later with pertussis vaccination; whooping cough catches up with them.

Difficult birth, perinatal problems, extended period in special care but no suspected brain damage

Most babies who have had difficult deliveries or a stormy period after birth should receive pertussis immunization but the doctor may need to be consulted. The recommendations for whooping cough immunization (p. 209) no longer exclude babies with a history of cerebral irritation in the neonatal period. If the baby seems to be developing normally at the time immunizations are due, pertussis should be given.

Suspected cerebral damage

If the baby is developing normally, pertussis should be given. If there is any substantial doubt over whether the child has sustained damage, **the nurse or doctor should seek advice from a paediatrician or other appropriate specialist (preferably by telephone) rather than deny the child protection against whooping cough or any other disease.**

It is often difficult to decide whether cerebral damage has taken place in babies whose stay in hospital following birth has been long and difficult. Some special-care baby units specify in their discharge summaries the immunizations that should be given. This practice is to be encouraged as not only is it helpful for primary-care staff, but also at the time first immunizations are due many families will still be attending hospital and will therefore pay close attention to the opinion of their hospital specialist. Where there is any doubt, neonatal units should give guidance over the phone to an enquiring doctor.

Documented cerebral damage

Documented cerebral damage is **not** a contraindication to pertussis immunization, and children with stable neurological conditions should be immunized with all indicated vaccines, including pertussis and MMR (see p. 209). Children who have suffered in the birth period also often have chronic lung disease (bronchopulmonary dysplasia) and hence are at particular risk from whooping cough disease. However, individual evaluation is required while the nature of the damage becomes clear. **Where the nurse or doctor is unsure as to whether to give pertussis or not they should seek advice from a paediatrician or other specialist (preferably by telephone) rather than deny the child protection.**

Premature babies—when should immunization start?

Immunizations start three months after birth no matter how premature the baby. All the evidence points to protection being just as effective as in the term infant. Some babies now begin immunization before they are discharged from neonatal units. When this is done the local immunization record holders must be informed.

Small babies

Immunizations start at three months after birth irrespective of weight. The smaller the baby or child the more they are at risk if whooping cough is caught.

Breastfeeding babies

Breastfeeding does not interfere with immunization (this includes polio drops). The same is true no matter what medication the mother is taking.

Babies and children with minor illnesses

Unwell babies and children

It is important to assess each case individually and particularly to ask about feeding and to take the temperature. If the illness is minimal or in the recovery phase, the child is feeding normally, and the temperature is under 37.5°C, immunization should proceed. If the parents feel their child is just starting an illness, it will be wiser to defer immunization for a week. The same applies for babies or children who are clearly unwell in the doctor's view. A useful rule is that children should not be immunized if their temperature is over 37.5°C and ill babies and children may need to be seen by a doctor for treatment of their illness. If in doubt, a medical opinion should be sought to ascertain fitness for immunization. One further useful rule used by nurses is that any baby or child whose immunizations have to be deferred on two successive weeks should see a doctor at, or as soon as possible after, the second occasion.

Babies who are snuffly or chesty

Some babies always seem a bit snuffly or chesty and others carry on coughing long after a respiratory illness. If the baby is apyrexial and feeding well, it is safe to ignore chronic snuffles, coughs, and wheezes, and proceed with immunization; otherwise such babies would never receive protection. Any child whose immunization is deferred on two successive weeks should be seen by a doctor.

Babies and children with a rash

As long as the baby or child is well and has no fever she can be immunized.

Babies and children who have had contact with an infectious illness recently

As long as the baby or child is well he can be immunized. This is particularly important for measles where a dose of MMR protects unimmunized children from the worst effects of the illness.

Babies and children with diarrhoea

If a baby or child is generally unwell with acute diarrhoea then all immunizations should be deferred for a week. In the essentially well individual diarrhoea is irrelevant to all injected immunizations and these should all be given. However, polio drops should be delayed unless there is substantial doubt whether the family will return, in which case a better strategy is to give the drops plus an extra dose at a later date. Some babies and children always have loose stools (toddler diarrhoea) and if such a child is well, give polio drops.

Babies and children reported to have already had an illness

Usually this is when the baby is supposed to have already had measles or whooping cough. Nurses should never tell parents that immunization will not be needed but must first consult the doctor. Many babies who are reported to have had measles (which is rare in the UK before the first birthday) or whooping cough have, in fact, had another illness with some resemblance to the rash of measles or the cough of whooping cough. Measles in particular is over-diagnosed: almost any rash will eventually be called measles if it is presented to enough people! Babies and children who are not immunized for this reason will probably catch the real illness later, and this is the principal way they may seem to have a disease twice. Even if they have actually had the illness, there is no extra risk from being immunized. Only positive serology is acceptable proof of measles infection and then the child must still have MMR to receive protection against mumps and rubella. A positive immunofluorescence test or culture of *Bordetella* is the only acceptable proof of *B. pertussis* infection. Girls with an alleged history of rubella should still be immunized in secondary school unless serology shows the girl to be immune. See also Parental counselling, p. 174.

BABIES AND CHILDREN ON ANTIBIOTICS AND OTHER MEDICINES

Babies and children on antibiotics

As long as they have almost recovered from their illness, it is acceptable to proceed with immunization. A nurse or community children's doctor may decide to first consult the GP who prescribed the medicine. Immunization works perfectly well and is just as safe for children on antibiotics.

Babies or children on other common medicines, e.g. nystatin elixir

Babies and children may be immunized as long as they are well.

Children and babies having steroids

This is only relevant for live vaccines (polio, MMR, BCG, and rubella—see list p. 258) and even then only in the rare circumstances where high doses of steroids are being given. The criteria are a course of injected or oral steroids of 2 mg/kg or more for over one continuous week in the preceding three months. Shorter courses, lower doses, and locally acting preparations (e.g. inhaled Becotide and topical skin steroids) do not interfere with immunization.

Previous reactions

Babies and children who have had a previous severe reaction to a vaccine which included pertussis

If the next indicated immunization contains pertussis, check whether the reaction meets the criteria given. The definition of a severe reaction is:

Local: An extensive area of redness at the vaccination site which becomes indurated (hard) and involves most of the front and side of the thigh, or a major part of the circumference of the upper arm.

General: Fever over 39.5°C occurring within 48 hours, or any one of the following occurring within 72 hours, of an immunization: anaphylaxis, bronchospasm (wheeze), laryngeal oedema, generalized collapse, prolonged unresponsiveness, convulsions, prolonged inconsolable screaming.

On the uncommon occasion where the reaction meets these criteria pertussis should be excluded from future injections. This must be documented and the reaction recorded and reported (see p. 183).

Where parents have experienced less severe reactions in their child they may find counselling from a well-informed doctor useful. Where a reaction has been less than that described, or the immunizing nurse or doctor is unsure whether it fits the criteria, they should never advise immunizing with just diphtheria and tetanus. They should seek advice from a paediatrician or other appropriate specialist (preferably by phone) rather than deny the child protection. See also Parental Counselling, p. 174.

FITS, FEBRILE CONVULSIONS, DEVELOPMENTAL DELAY, NEUROLOGICAL DISEASE, CEREBRAL PALSY

Babies and children who have had fits or febrile convulsions

Parents may call temper tantrums, breath-holding attacks, rigors, or faints 'fits'. There are also many different kinds of fits, some more relevant to immunization than others (see next paragraph). A personal history of fits is no longer a contraindication to pertussis immunization, and children with stable neurological conditions, such as epilepsy, may be vaccinated (see p. 209). Hence most babies or children who have had fits can be immunized with pertussis vaccine. Parents of such children are usually anxious about immunization and these are circumstances where cases require individual evaluation by the doctor with the parents. Fits are no reason for denying a child MMR, but precautions may be needed to prevent or deal with any febrile reactions (see p. 203). Parents whose child has had a febrile convulsion need reminding that their child is especially likely to have another if it catches measles and so immunization with MMR is especially important. Fits are not relevant to other immunizations. If the family is being cared for by a paediatrician it will be wise to agree on a joint community/hospital immunization policy.

Babies and children who had **neonatal fits** due to hypocalcaemia can certainly be immunized with pertussis vaccine. The same applies for children whose fits were due to hypoglycaemia or hypoxia where the child did not sustain damage.

Babies and children with mild developmental delay

All immunizations including pertussis and MMR may be given. It is important that the parents understand about their child's delay before immunization commences.

Babies and children with serious developmental delay

Most children with severe developmental delay should not be denied protection, including that of pertussis and MMR vaccine. If the condition is stable (e.g. in established cerebral palsy), then immunization should be given. Other cases will, however, need assessment, and where a paediatrician is already involved she or he should be contacted first. This particularly applies if the underlying cause of the delay is undiagnosed. Such assessment is best anticipated prior to any immunization being due.

Neurological disease

Most of these children will be under the care of a paediatrician who should be consulted. For progressive cerebral disease, such as neurodegenerative conditions (**but not muscular dystrophy**), it would seem reasonable to omit pertussis, while polio, diphtheria, tetanus, and MMR vaccines should be given as usual (see also next paragraph).

Stable neurological conditions (cerebral palsy, spina bifida, hydrocephalus, etc.)

The child should be given pertussis immunization as well as all other indicated vaccines (taking precautions for MMR if the child has had fits). It will be advisable to contact the child's paediatrician prior to immunization to ensure a consistent policy.

Non-neurological illness

The baby or child with long-term chest or heart condition (e.g. cystic fibrosis or congenital heart disease)

It is particularly important that these children are protected with pertussis and MMR. The normal criteria for fitness to immunize (see p. 241) should be used. Where the child is chronically or usually unwell (e.g. the cyanotic child) immunization must not be put off without consulting the doctor. The latter will need to bear in mind that to prevent deterioration of their condition as a result of whooping cough or measles such children may need to be immunized when in a state of chronic ill health. Older children with cystic fibrosis may benefit from annual influenza immunization.

Immunodeficient children

See p. 258.

Down's syndrome, simple mental retardation

As for stable neurological conditions, these children are entitled to all the usual immunizations. Some children with Down's seem especially vulnerable to respiratory infections and are constantly snuffly or chesty, and this is not a contraindication to immunization.

Babies and children with asthma, eczema, hay fever, or simple allergies

All routine immunizations should be given, including whooping cough and MMR.

The child with extreme or severe egg allergy

For MMR or monovalent measles this is only important in the extremely rare circumstances when the allergy is extreme to the point of anaphylaxis, in which case further advice should be sought prior to immunization with these vaccines. For the less commonly given vaccinations of influenza and yellow fever, severe egg allergy is a contraindication. All other routine protection should be given and the commoner forms of egg allergy (diarrhoea, skin rashes) are of no importance.

FAMILY HISTORY

Mother or father, brother or sister[*] have had fits

These children should have all immunizations, including whooping cough and MMR. If the fits are due to idiopathic epilepsy, a doctor should counsel the parents concerning management of the child after immunization as there is a very small additional risk of a febrile convulsion (see MMR, p. 203).

See also Parental Counselling, p. 174.

---

[*]These are sometimes referred to as first-degree relatives.

Grandparents, aunts, uncles, fifth cousins, etc. having fits

Any fits in relatives beyond the immediate (first-degree) family are irrelevant to immunization. The child can receive all immunizations without special precautions.

Family history of neurological disease

There is no additional risk. All immunizations should be given.

A brother or sister had a severe immunization reaction

All immunizations should be given; however, parents may understandably be nervous and need to consult the doctor before proceeding. See also Parental counselling, p. 174.

Family history of asthma, eczema, hay fever, or allergies

These are all irrelevant to immunization. The baby or child should be given full protection.

Administrative problems

Interrupted immunization course

In this case the immunizer should give the next immunization that the child is due to receive. If more than one is overdue (for example Triple, polio, and MMR), then all should be given at the same session. However, if more than one Triple is overdue they still need to be spaced apart at the usual intervals.

It is never necessary to restart an immunization course.

Pre-school booster—prior injections overdue

When children come for their pre-school booster it often turns out that they have missed out on some immunizations. Children should catch up with these on this occasion. A classical story is a child who presents at booster time having only had two Triples (DTP) and polios. She or he should have the third Triple, the MMR, and polio at one visit. They will then need the diphtheria/tetanus and polio boosters in three years' time. **If only the measles has been missed, the pre-school booster is given at the usual time with the MMR in the other arm.**

Pre-school booster—measles already given

The child should be given MMR as well as the diphtheria/tetanus and polio booster.

Older children behind in immunization

If over three but under 10 years old, the child should have any immunizations missed including MMR (up to the sixteenth birthday). This includes pertussis as this child will place any younger children (especially babies) at risk if he or she catches whooping cough. The immunizations can be given at monthly intervals (see p. 313 for detailed schedules).

If over 10 years old, the child should have any immunizations that have been missed. If diphtheria is needed, the special adult vaccine is required; alternatively a one-fifth dose (0.1 ml) of the normal vaccine can be given. There is no need for a Schick test (a measurement of immunity to diphtheria). It is important to remember to ask if the child has already had a tetanus injection at casualty or from a general practitioner.

Giving two immunizations at once

It is acceptable to give immunizations simultaneously, including the live vaccines (polio, MMR, rubella, and BCG). **However, it is**

important never to mix vaccines in the same syringe. If giving two injections, it is good practice to give one in each arm and to document this so that it is possible to attribute any local reaction to the correct vaccine.

Once one live vaccine has been given it is usually recommended to wait three weeks before giving another. However, the evidence that this is of any clinical importance is weak, and where two live vaccines are inadvertently given within the time period it is not justified to repeat either. When BCG is given it is recommended to allow three months to elapse before giving any other vaccination in the same arm, as this has been associated with painful lymph nodes under the arm.

Child due for routine immunization who has recently had a tetanus injection

It is simplest to ignore the tetanus and proceed with the indicated immunization.

Children of pregnant mothers

All immunizations should be given, including polio.

Recent immigrants

It can be difficult to find out what immunizations have been given to immigrants, and it may be necessary to treat the children and the rest of the family as if they were unimmunized and start a complete programme (see p. 313 for schedules). It is particularly important to check the rubella serology of any young women in the family and to give rubella vaccine if necessary. A Heaf or Mantoux test is always needed if the family has come from an area with high levels of tuberculosis (India, Bangladesh, Pakistan, East Asia, Africa, and other Third World countries).

Non-English speaking parents

An interpreter is mandatory for taking a history. Simply obtaining a signature without proper counselling is bad practice.

Children from another area with inadequate records

To wait for full details from another district can mean an intolerable delay and such children should not be denied protection. It is wise to involve a doctor in deciding on immunization, not least as the children may have other medical or developmental problems needing assessment and treatment.

Unknown family history, fostered or adopted babies and children

While efforts should be made to obtain a family history, it is worth noting that only fits in parents or siblings are relevant. The probability of familial epilepsy is small, which anyway is only a special consideration (for pertussis and MMR) of very low risk. Where the history is unobtainable, the case should be considered by a doctor. The chances of the child catching measles or whooping cough are high and therefore the risks arising from leaving the child unprotected are considerably higher than from any immunization.

Children in care

Written permission has to be given by the appropriate member of the Social Services Department for children to enter a course of immunizations. Care needs to be taken in getting a reliable history concerning previous immunizations and any severe reaction. This will need pointing out to Social Services so that when the child comes for immunization they are accompanied by someone who can provide such a history.

Wards of court

Written permission will need to be sought from the Court. This can take months and should be thought about well before immunizations are due. As for children in care, a reliable history concerning previous immunizations should be obtained if at all possible.

Mothers under 16

The mother is usually the person to give any written consent. Special care should be taken to ensure counselling is adequate.

Person accompanying the baby or child scarcely knows them

It should be parents or guardians who give any necessary written consent for entering an immunization programme. For subsequent injections the person who brings the child needs to know him well enough to give a proper history about reactions to previous immunizations and also to judge whether the child is currently well.

OTHER PROBLEMS

Babies who vomit after polio drops

This is only important if the baby has a substantial vomit in the first hour after immunization, in which case more drops should be given.

Blood transfusion

A child who has recently had a transfusion can be immunized. It is unusual for children to need transfusions and it will be sensible to ask the reason for this so as to check that the child does not have an immunodeficient state (e.g. leukaemia) that necessitated the transfusion. It is suggested that blood transfusion may interfere with rubella immunization. This eventuality most commonly arises in the postnatal seronegative woman who had a transfusion and needs immunization. This can be given when three months have elapsed.

General anaesthetic

Any child may have a mild reaction to an immunization and this could complicate an anaesthetic. Hence immunization should be avoided in the three days (12 days for MMR) before an anaesthetic for a pre-arranged operation. Children can have any immunization needed as soon as they are over an anaesthetic, and there is no reason to believe any anaesthetic prevents immunization working. There is no reason for putting off routine surgery outside of these time limits and an urgently needed operation should proceed irrespective of recent immunizations.

AFTER INJURY

Severe injuries

Burns or wounds with the following features require emergency treatment, including consideration for protection against tetanus: a significant amount of dead tissue; or a puncture-type wound; or soiling with earth or other material likely to be contaminated with tetanus; or obvious evidence of infection; or any wound where there has been more than six hours before receiving surgical treatment; or a human or animal bite.

The wound should be cleaned and the child given anti-tetanus protection according to the following schedule.

1. **Children (or adults) not known to have completed a full course of tetanus injections** (the number of tetanus injections will depend on the age of the child: a one-year-old should have had three injections, a five-year-old four injections, etc.) and **children (or adults) who had their last tetanus injection more than 10 years previously** should all have anti-tetanus immunoglobulin by intramuscular injection in one limb and the first of a

course of three tetanus injections in the other limb. The remaining tetanus injections are given at monthly intervals or (for the child under three years of age) as per the national schedule.

2. **Children (or adults) who have only had a single injection** should be treated as (1) with anti-tetanus immunoglobulin and an immediate tetanus injection but they will only need one more tetanus injection later.

3. **Children (or adults) who completed a primary course (three injections) or had a booster within 5–10 years beforehand** should not have immunoglobulin and need only be given a single tetanus injection.

4. **Children (or adults) who completed a primary course or had a booster within the last five years** should not have immunoglobulin and should only receive a booster if the doctor judges the risk of tetanus to be high.

Less severe injuries

If the wound is less severe than listed above, a child midway through a primary immunization course does not need a booster (for example, a nine-month-old with a minor scratch who has had two DTP immunizations). Some doctors may prefer to give a tetanus toxoid injection in casualty, especially if only one immunization has been given, as the protection afforded by this is low. If this is done, the local health authority and the child's general practitioner must be notified. An alternative (and preferable) strategy is simply to give the next DTP and polio at the time of the injury.

Immunization and protection of infants and children with specific problems

Many of the children covered below will be under the care of both hospital specialists and general practitioners. Early consultation is recommended to ensure agreement on immunization policy. Nothing is more confusing for parents than to receive differing advice and if this occurs the child is usually denied protection. When a normal immunization schedule is recommended this is as per the national schedule (on back cover).

Achondroplasia/hypochondroplasia—normal immunization schedule.

AIDS—see HIV infection (p. 257).

Allergy—a history of allergy eczema or asthma is not a contraindication to immunization. Where there has been an anaphylactic response to eggs, MMR (measles/mumps/rubella), influenza, and yellow fever should not be given without specialist advice (see p. 270).

Asplenia—pneumococcal vaccine is recommended in addition to normal schedules. Vaccine alone will not give complete protection against pneumococcal disease, particularly in children with sickle-cell disease where extra protection with oral penicillin is necessary. Penicillin is a safe precaution in children following splenectomy for trauma or hereditary spherocytosis.

Arthritis—see juvenile rheumatoid arthritis.

Asthma—normal immunization schedule. If very severe, consider influenza immunization.

Birth asphyxia—normal schedule in absence of fits or developmental delay. Infants with early neonatal fits following asphyxia come into the 'problem history' group (see p. 209) for pertussis. The presence of bronchopulmonary dysplasia/chronic lung disease is a strong indication for pertussis immunization.

Cerebral palsy—normal schedule if stable; if history of seizures, advise on temperature control (see p. 209).

Congenital heart disease—normal immunization schedule. Consider influenza immunization for children with cyanotic heart disease over six months of age. See also endocarditis prophylaxis, p. 260.

Cystic fibrosis—normal immunization schedule. Annual influenza vaccination is recommended in children over six months.

Diabetes mellitus—normal immunization schedule.

Down's syndrome—normal immunization schedule.

Endocarditis prophylaxis—see p. 260.

Endocrine disorders—normal immunization schedule.

Epilepsy—see febrile convulsions.

Febrile convulsions—pertussis immunization is normally completed before these develop. However, where they have occurred, or immunization has been delayed, pertussis vaccine should be given (see p. 209) and MMR. Immunoglobulin should **not** be used and parents should be advised on temperature control.

Growth hormone deficiency—normal immunization schedule.

Haemophilia and other non-malignant bleeding problems— normal immunization schedule. Give all injections subcutaneously (or intradermally if indicated) **not** intramuscularly.

Heart disease—see congenital heart disease (p. 257).

Human immunodeficiency virus (HIV)—all these children will be under the care of a specialist who should be consulted for discussion of an appropriate immunization course.

1. HIV-positive but asymptomatic children, including those of indeterminate status (HIV-positive children under 15 months where the reason for positivity may be passive transfer of maternal antibody), should receive the normal immunization schedule including: polio, diphtheria, pertussis, tetanus, MMR/ measles, rubella. BCG should **not** be given. Inactivated polio (IPV) may be given to a child when there is the risk of a parent being immunodepressed.

2. Symptomatic HIV-positive children will need to have their cases individually evaluated but, on the whole, they may be

given live virus vaccines (except BCG) as the benefits of protection outweigh the risks from the vaccines, especially where the diseases against which the children are being protected are prevalent. They should receive all appropriate inactivated vaccines.

Hydrocephalus—normal immunization schedule. In the presence of fits special consideration for pertussis immunization should be given (see p. 209) and MMR (see p. 203).

Immunodeficient/Immunodepressed—This state may follow disease or treatment. The following groups of children should not receive live vaccines (p. 163). For HIV infection see p. 37.

(1)   patients receiving high-dose corticosteroids (e.g. 2 mg/kg for more than a week), or immunosuppressive treatment including general irradiation; those suffering from malignant conditions such as lymphoma, leukaemia, Hodgkin's disease, or other tumours of the reticuloendothelial system; patients with impaired immunological mechanism as, for example, in hypogammaglobulinaemia;

(2)   children with immunosuppression from disease or therapy (e.g. in remission from acute leukaemia) until at least six months after chemotherapy has finished;

(3)   children treated with systemic corticosteroids at high dose (2 mg/kg/day for more than a week) until at least three months after treatment has stopped (children on lower daily doses of systemic corticosteroids for less than two weeks, and those who have moved onto either continuously lower doses or alternate day regimens for longer periods, may be given live virus vaccines).

All inactivated vaccines may be given to immunodepressed children. Immunodepressed children and their close contacts (siblings, class-mates, close friends) must be immunized with MMR. Measles has killed many immunodepressed children. **Community paediatricians and nurses bear a special responsibility to see that MMR uptake is particularly high in any school or day-care facility where**

Erratum

The sentence five lines from the bottom of page 258 should read:

The close contacts (siblings, class-mates, close friends) of immunodepressed children **must** be immunized with MMR.

such children are placed. There is no risk of virus transmission following measles, mumps, or rubella vaccines. Oral poliomyelitis vaccine (OPV) should not be given to these children, their siblings or other household contacts; inactivated vaccine (IPV) should be used in its place. In the case of malignancies, a complete immunization history is needed at the time of diagnosis and historical and serological evidence sought for immunity to measles, chickenpox, and rubella. Where either suggest non-immunity, children in categories (1) and (2) above will need an injection of immunoglobulin as soon as possible after exposure to measles or chickenpox. The specialist team looking after them must be contacted **immediately** such exposure is suspected. Children with congenital immune deficiencies may not respond to vaccines and some need regular doses of immunoglobulin. Children who develop chickenpox should be treated with acyclovir.

Juvenile rheumatoid arthritis—check rubella serology in girls and if negative immunize; delay if in active stage of disease.

Leukaemia—see immunodepressed.

Malabsorption—normal immunization schedule including oral polio.

Malignancies—see immunodepressed.

Meningitis—normal immunization schedule.

Metabolic disorders—many may receive the normal immunization schedule. This is, however, such a range of disorders, with some children in delicate metabolic states, that individual cases should be discussed with their supervising doctor.

Muscular dystrophy—normal immunization schedule.

Nephrotic syndrome—see immunodepressed.

Pregnancy—live vaccines are to be avoided unless the risk is high. Examples are women travelling to areas where polio or yellow fever is endemic. Inadvertent rubella immunization is not an indication for termination.

Prematurity—normal schedule for all immunizations given at appropriate times from birth.

Sickle-cell disease—see asplenia.

Spina bifida—normal immunization schedule.

Splenectomy—see asplenia.

Steroids—see immunodepressed.

Thalassaemia—see asplenia.

Toddler diarrhoea—normal immunization schedule, including oral polio.

Tonsillectomy, adenoidectomy, etc.—normal immunization schedule, including oral polio.

Turner's syndrome—normal immunization schedule.

ENDOCARDITIS PROPHYLAXIS FOR CHILDREN WITH HEART DEFECTS

Children with congenital heart defects are at risk from bacterial endocarditis caused by the transient bacteraemia released by certain dental and surgical procedures involving mucosa and infected tissue. They should be protected by antibiotic prophylaxis.

At particular risk are children with prosthetic heart valves or systemic to pulmonary artery shunts, but bacterial endocarditis should be considered when any child with a heart abnormality develops an unexplained febrile illness, especially if it follows a dental or surgical operation.

Parents should be told about the importance of high standards of oral hygiene and regular dental inspections for their children. It is helpful if they can be given brief written instructions about antibiotic prophylaxis to which they can refer when necessary or draw to the attention of dentists and surgeons at the appropriate times.

Prophylaxis should continue after the surgical repair of most heart defects but for a few the risk of endocarditis is so small that antibiotics are not recommended. These include: (a) repaired ostium secundium atrial septal defects (after six months); (b) closed patent ductus arteriosus.

For general dental treatment likely to cause gum bleeding, especially for extractions

The following should be given one hour before the procedure: amoxycillin 3.0 g orally to children over 10 years, and 1.5 g orally to children under 10; or, if there is an allergy to penicillin, erythromycin 1.0 g orally to children over 10 years and 0.5 g orally to children under 10. Note: these doses are 'rounded off' for convenience to suit children of school age likely to need dental treatment without general anaesthesia.

For procedures in hospital with a general anaesthetic

The following should be given intravenously with induction of anaesthesia:

1. Dental and respiratory tract surgery: amoxycillin 50 mg/kg.

2. Gastrointestinal and genitourinary surgery: amoxycillin 50 mg/ kg plus gentamicin 2 mg/kg. Note: if there is penicillin allergy, replace amoxycillin with erythromicin 20 mg/kg (as lactobionate) given slowly.

3. Children with prosthetic heart valves (at special risk): gentamicin 2 mg/kg plus vancomycin 20 mg/kg given slowly.

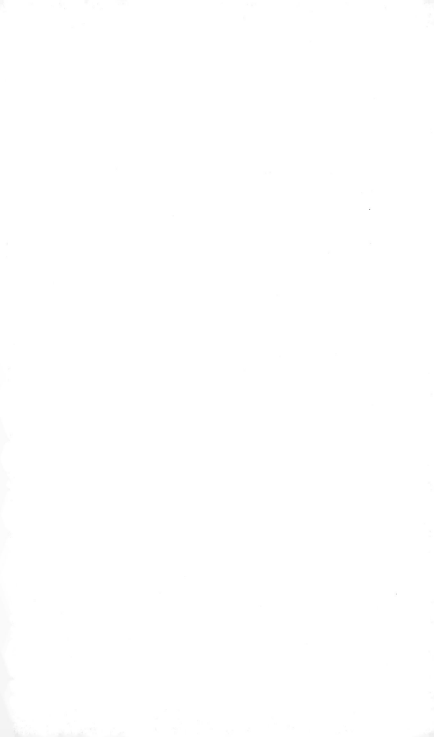

Travel Abroad

Travel abroad

International travel is increasing: in 1979 UK residents made 14 million trips abroad; by 1986 the figure was 23 million, 12 per cent to destinations beyond Europe.

Most children travelling abroad fall into one of two major groups: (a) those taking a holiday in Europe and the Mediterranean; and (b) those returning with their parents to the countries of origin, of which the Indian subcontinent (ISC) is the most common, followed by West Africa. In addition, smaller numbers undertake more ambitious trips and travel advice may be needed for children visiting almost any country in the world.

The infections to which a child may be exposed include those commoner in less-developed countries, many of which are amenable to immunization or chemoprophylaxis (e.g. typhoid, polio, diphtheria, yellow fever, malaria) and also those which remain prevalent in Britain (gastroenteritis, whooping cough, hepatitis, measles, tuberculosis). With air travel, almost all diseases contracted abroad may be incubating on return. Hence, a history of recent travel must be sought in any child with fever, gastrointestinal, or other symptoms suggestive of infection.

Health advice for travel is a complex subject and a text can never be up to date. Also, the protection recommended for an extended stay may be very different from that for a holiday. This section simply outlines the advice most commonly sought and lists the sources which the health-care worker or traveller can consult for more detailed and current information (see also Further reading, p. 332.)

General advice

Travel abroad has many potential hazards, not all associated with infection. These include different safety standards, exposure to extremes of climate, and language difficulties all compounding ignorance of the local medical system. To a certain extent, parents must exercise their own common sense regarding their child's visit. A family checklist is: appropriate clothing, entertainment for the journey, adequate protection against sunburn, medical insurance, immunization prophylaxis, and simple medications.

These topics are well covered in many popular and professional publications, two examples of which are listed in Further reading nos 11 and 12 (p. 332). Specific guidelines for individual countries are also provided in the DHSS leaflet *Protect your health abroad* (Further reading, no. 13) which is updated annually and available on Prestel, page 50063.

Simple precautions

Eighty per cent of holiday-acquired infections (mostly the various forms of gastroenteritis) are water and/or food borne, and though they are not preventable by immunization, simple precautions will help to protect all family members. Some guidelines are given below. The extent to which they are followed will depend on local conditions and family preference. However, it is wise to emphasize to parents that diarrhoea is a common cause of a spoilt holiday and may be a serious risk.

1. Scrupulous attention to hand hygiene especially after using the toilet, nappy-changing, and before meals. Soap and/or toilet paper may be unavailable locally.

2. Where the water supply may be of uncertain quality (that is most countries outside northern Europe, North America, New Zealand, Australia, and urban South Africa), the traveller should not drink water from taps or other sources. Hot, bottled, or canned drinks with well-known brand names are safest. Alternatively, water can be treated. If visible matter is present, the water should first be strained through a closely woven cloth. Sterilization is achieved by boiling for five minutes or disinfecting. Appropriate disinfectants are chlorine and iodine (either liquid bleach, tincture of iodine, or 'sterilizing' tablets). Iodine is preferable as chlorine is less effective. All tablets have makers'

instructions. Tincture of iodine (2 per cent) should be used at a concentration of 4 drops to 1 litre of water; the water is then allowed to stand for 30 minutes before use.

3. In the same countries as those where water precautions are advised the following should be avoided: raw vegetables, salads, unpeeled fruit, raw shellfish, cream, ice-cream, under-done meat or fish, uncooked or cold pre-cooked food, and ice cubes. Similarly, unpasteurized milk (unless boiled) and cheese apart from that known to be made from pasteurized milk, may also carry infection.

4. Self-caterers should cook meat well. Fruit and vegetables should be washed thoroughly in clean soapy water. If they are not then being cooked, they should be soaked for half an hour in treated water at three times the concentration of disinfectant used for purifying drinking water (see above).

5. In case a child develops gastroenteritis, the family need to pack some oral rehydration mixture (e.g. Dioralyte, Rehidrat). One cupful for each loose stool is a memorable dosage but parents must seek medical help if excessive vomiting, severe diarrhoea, drowsiness, or other signs of dehydration occur, especially in a young baby (see p. 58).

6. Children (and adults) should not play on beaches or swim in water visibly polluted with sewage.

SPECIFIC ADVICE FOR PARTICULAR COUNTRIES AND DISEASES

Information sources

Because the specific advice can change so frequently, it is best for the traveller or the professional either to consult regularly updated publications or to contact designated information centres. The former are: the DHSS pamphlet *Protect your health abroad* (Further reading, no. 13); the WHO booklet *Vaccination certificate require-*

ments and health advice for international travel (Further reading,
no. 14); and the medical newspaper *Pulse* (table updated monthly).
All these list the advice and requirements by country. However, the
advice is not always consistent. Requirements tend to lag behind the
times (until recently a few countries still needed proof of smallpox
immunization!) and protection in addition to the formal requirements is frequently advisable. Also, what is necessary for a brief trip
to a country's main city may be very different from the protection
appropriate for an extended stay up-country. The main information
centres are listed in Appendix 5 (p. 315) and a more detailed list of
specialist associations is provided in *Travellers' health* (Further
reading, no. 11).

Parents taking children on a complicated tour or extended trip
may find the Medical Advisory Services for Travellers Abroad
(MASTA) useful. Based at the London School of Hygiene and
Tropical Medicine, it tailors a personalized health brief to the
specific journey and medical history (see Appendix 5, p. 315 for
address). It does charge a fee. Family application forms are available
from MASTA and most branches of Boots.

ROUTINE IMMUNIZATIONS FOR TRAVEL

Polio

There have recently been several cases of poliomyelitis in the
children of African and Asian immigrant parents. Although born in
Britain, they had either not started or completed their immunization
before being taken on visits to the home country. It cannot be
assumed that a course will be completed abroad. The vaccine may
not be available, and some parents do not realize the need for
continuing the course. Hence, such high-risk babies and children
must be fully protected before they leave, either by using an
accelerated programme of immunization at monthly intervals (see p.
313) or even by starting in the neonatal period. It is equally
important to advise that children of any age visiting an endemic area
(for practical purposes all less-developed countries) should be fully

immunized against polio. Adults accompanying them should have boosters if they have had none in the preceding 10 years.

Diphtheria, measles

Both are common in the ISC and Africa. All British children should be protected by ensuring immunization is up to date. No booster will be needed for fully immunized children or adults. Children going to the USA and entering school or registered day-care will be required by law to produce documentary proof of immunization, including MMR.

Tuberculosis

Children at risk are those making extended visits to developing countries. If the child has not had BCG as a neonate, it must be given before visiting an endemic area for a month or more. Forward planning is needed as a Heaf or Mantoux test must be used first and six weeks should elapse between BCG and departure.

Tetanus

Whatever and wherever the holiday, the consultation for advice should include ensuring up-to-date tetanus vaccination (NB: not more frequently than 10-yearly after the primary course).

ADDITIONAL IMMUNIZATIONS AND CHEMOPROPHYLAXIS COMMONLY RECOMMENDED FOR TRAVEL

Typhoid

There are between 50 and 60 notifications of typhoid in children each year in England and Wales, the majority acquired overseas, chiefly in the ISC. Prevention is most effectively achieved by good standards of personal hygiene and avoidance of contaminated food and water (see p. 278). A vaccine is available but is only moderately protective and its effectiveness wanes rapidly (see p. 267).

Cholera

This disease is endemic in the ISC with epidemics in Africa, the Middle East, and occasionally the Mediterranean. A handful of cases occur annually in the UK, all acquired abroad. As for typhoid, good hygiene is the best prevention (see p. 144) and the vaccine is of very limited effectiveness (see p. 230).

Yellow fever

This disease occurs in two endemic zones, Central Africa and the northern zone of South America, with cases occurring in both urban and rural settings. Cases are almost unheard of in Britain but travellers to these countries are certainly at risk and must be protected. In addition, many countries require the immunization which is used in two situations: (a) for travellers to the endemic zones; and (b) for travellers to non-endemic areas which require evidence of immunity from visitors who have passed through an endemic zone *en route* (these countries have climates and mosquitos which would favour transmission, hence they wish to prevent disease introduction). See *Protect your health abroad* (Further reading, no. 13) for a current list of the centres offering immunization. For a description of the disease, see p. 152; and of the immunization, see p. 233.

Malaria

(See also p. 88.) In 1986 British families made 1.2 million trips to endemic areas: Africa, including the Mediterranean coast; the Indian subcontinent; the tropical Far East; South and Central America, plus Haiti (see p. 273 for a full list). Asian or African parents are often unaware of the need for chemoprophylaxis and, consequently, now make up half the cases reported in the UK. Often their home area was relatively free from malaria when they lived there, or they may believe that their childhood immunity should still protect them. The latter is certainly untrue, and families must be persuaded of the importance of prevention. There are three approaches to prevention of malaria and travel advice must include **all** of these.

Avoidance of mosquito bites

These are most likely after sunset and indoors.

1. It is recommended to sleep under a mosquito net (available from MASTA (see Appendix 5, p. 317); nets are priced £25–32), preferably one impregnated with an insecticide such as permethrin (Perigen–manufactured by Wellcome as a 10 per cent solution). The edges of the net must be tucked under the mattress during daylight hours, ensuring that no mosquitoes are trapped inside. A needle and thread should be packed as these nets invariably sustain tears.

2. Accommodation with mosquito screening on windows and doors is desirable and it is necessary to be meticulous about closing these screens, especially from late afternoon on. Spraying the rooms with a knock-down insecticide at this time will eliminate any determined invaders who have breached the defences.

3. When out of doors in the evening all family members should wear clothes which cover arms and legs, to reduce the amount of exposed skin. A mosquito repellent such as diethyl toluamide (DEET) is also worth spreading on the skin.

Chemoprophylaxis

The main antimalarials are shown in Table 14, and these may be bought without prescription in some countries. Amodiaquine and Fansidar are no longer recommended for prophylaxis because of serious side-effects. Pyrimethamine on its own (Daraprim) must **not** be used as it seems particularly ineffective in preventing severe falciparum malaria.

Table 14 Malaria prophylaxis

Name	Adult prophylactic dose
Chloroquine (Nivaquine, Avloclor)	300 mg base (2 tablets) weekly
Proguanil (Paludrine)	200 mg (2 tablets) daily
Maloprim (pyrimethamine 12.5 mg + dapsone 100 mg)	1 tablet weekly

Doses for children are (all given at same intervals as for adults):

	Proguanil/chloroquine	Maloprim
Under 6 weeks	One-eighth adult dose	Not recommended
6 weeks to 11 months	Quarter adult dose	One-eighth adult dose
1–5 years	Half adult dose	Quarter adult dose
6–11 years	Three-quarters adult dose	Half adult dose
Over 12 years	Adult dose	Adult dose

Determining the most appropriate regimen for a family is not straightforward. Factors include area of travel, length of stay, and local drug resistance. In such circumstances it is best to consult one of the national advice centres (see Appendix 5). However, it is not recommended to 'shop around' as experts may differ on what is the best regime even in specific circumstances. Medication should be started one week before leaving the UK, be continued throughout the stay in the area, and for **4–6 weeks after return**.

Countries with malaria are classified by the recommended regimes A–C. Within each area or category countries are listed by whether chloroquine-resistant falciparum malaria is present, and arranged by continent. The symbol (p) following a country indicates that substantial areas are malaria-free, and (s) indicates a substantial degree of seasonal malaria absence. The WHO booklet on *Vaccination requirements for international travel* (Further reading, no. 14) for the current year should be consulted for details of areas within countries (p) and months when malaria transmission (s) occurs.

Regime A: proguanil and chloroquine

(1) All sub-Saharan Africa:

(a) with chloroquine resistance: Angola, Burkina Faso, Burundi, Cameroon, Comoros, Congo, Equatorial Guinea, Ethiopia, Gabon, Ghana, Guinea-Bissau, Kenya, Madagascar, Malawi, Mozambique, Namibia (p), Senegal, Rwanda, South Africa (p) (s), Sudan, Tanzania, Uganda, Zaire, Zambia, Zimbabwe;

(b) without chloroquine resistance (many of these areas are expected to become chloroquine resistant): Benin, Botswana (p) (s), Central Africa Republic, Chad, Djibouti, Gambia, Guinea, Ivory Coast, Liberia, Mali, Mauritania, Niger, Nigeria, Sao Tome and Principe, Sierra Leone, Somalia, Swaziland, Togo;

(2) Asia: Bhutan, Iran;

(3) South Asia and China (with chloroquine resistance): Bangladesh, China (p) (s), India, Nepal, Pakistan, Sri Lanka;

(4) Latin America (with chloroquine resistance): Bolivia, Brazil (p), Columbia, Ecuador, French Guiana, Guyana, Panama, Peru, Surinam, Venezuela (p).

Regime B: Maloprim and chloroquine

Southeast Asia and Oceania: Burma, Kampuchea, Indonesia, Laos, Malaysia (p), Thailand, Vietnam, Phillipines (p), Papua New Guinea, Solomon Islands, Vanuatu. (Major cities of Southeast Asia are usually malaria-free.)

Regime C: Proguanil

(1) Asia: Afghanistan, Iraq (p), Maldives (p), Mauritius (p), North Yemen, Oman, Saudi Arabia (p), South Yemen, Syria (s), Turkey (p) (s), United Arab Emirates (p);

(2) Americas: Argentina (p) (s), Belize, Costa Rica (p), Dominican Republic, El Salvador, Guatemala, Haiti, Honduras, Mexico (p), Nicaragua, Paraguay (p);

(3) North Africa: Algeria (p) (s), Egypt (p) (s), Libya (p) (s), Morocco (p) (s).

Management of fever

It is important to stress to families that protection is **not** absolute. Parents should point out to the doctor the details of their travels, even if they occurred several years earlier. If the family is going to a very remote area far from medical help, they should contact one of the Advice Centres regarding advice on self-administered treatment regimes. Two recommended courses for areas covered by regimes A and B are:

Areas covered by Regime A

Fansidar: one tablet contains 500 mg sulfadoxine, 25 mg pyrimethamine; adult dose is 3 tablets taken together once only. Reduce adult dose as per Maloprim.

Areas covered by Regime B, and East Africa

Quinine: adult dose is 600 mg (2 tablets) every 8 hours for 5 days (30 tablets in total).

Prophylactics should be continued throughout the attack and subsequently. Self-medication is, however, to be avoided if medical help is accessible, and the prescribing doctor should warn about the principal side-effects of all these drugs. Proguanil: mild stomach upsets; chloroquine: mild stomach upsets and headaches; Maloprim: minimal; Fansidar: skin reactions and stomach upsets; other effects are rare with short therapeutic doses. Parents should be advised that all these medicines can be given mixed in jam or other disguisers of taste. Chloroquine has a particularly bitter taste.

Hepatitis A

Rates of this infection are highest in travellers returning from Asia and Africa, although anyone consuming impure water or unhygienically prepared food in any country, or living in crowded conditions, is at risk.

Protection

Advise against consumption of high hepatitis-risk shellfish (e.g. mussels, cockles, oysters) on holiday. Human normal immunoglobulin (HNIG) is highly effective at preventing infection, and dosages for children for protection lasting three or six months are given on p. 76. However, hepatitis in very young children is mild, indeed often asymptomatic, so it is unusual to give HNIG to travellers under five. Children (and adults) who repeatedly go to developing countries should have their immunity checked—they may already be immune and can be spared repeated injections. HNIG should be given just before departure and this can cause problems in travellers who present late for their immunoprophylaxis, as it may interfere with immunizations. It is usually advised that HNIG is not given until two weeks after a live virus vaccine, to avoid its reducing the immune response. It has, however, been shown that both individuals who already have some polio immunity (and probably those who don't) and those susceptible to yellow fever mount an adequate response to these vaccines even if HNIG is given simultaneously or up to a week after.

Hepatitis B
See p. 194.

IMMUNIZATIONS LESS COMMONLY REQUIRED

Rabies

Three of six cases of imported human rabies between 1977 and 1987 were children, all bitten by dogs in the ISC. Human diploid-cell rabies vaccine (HDCRV) containing inactivated virus is highly effective when administered either pre- or post-exposure and has few side-effects. However, pre-exposure rabies prophylaxis is not routinely recommended for travellers, even those visiting highly endemic zones such as the ISC, Africa, and Latin America. This is because the risk of being bitten by a rabid animal during a short stay is small and when it does occur post-exposure vaccination is highly effective. It should, however, be considered if a family or child is going to a high-risk area where the availability of post-exposure prophylaxis is in doubt. **Specialist consultation is required**. Two injections are needed one month apart and the vaccine is not available on the NHS. It can, however, be given intradermally so that two 1 ml vials (£17 in 1988) will cover a family of four. See p. 281 for details. **Information on this and post-exposure measures are available from Public Health Laboratories, departments of infectious disease, and the CDSC** (see Appendix 5, p. 315).

Whether or not pre-exposure vaccine is given, it is essential to educate parents about the risk of rabies which, without post-exposure immunization, is untreatable, causing an agonizing death in virtually 100 per cent of cases. The main risk is from bites, scratches, and licks from dogs, but also cats and any other mammal in the high-risk areas. Though rabies is endemic in other parts of the world, including Europe and North America, it is virtually completely confined to wild animals which normally have the good sense to stay away from children. Children must, however, be discouraged from approaching and handling both wild and domestic animals, especially in Asia and Africa and especially if they are wild cats and dogs. The advice for families is rather complex, as follows.

If a bite, lick, or scratch occurs from an animal that is behaving oddly or looking unwell, the wound must immediately be scrubbed with soap or detergent and running water for at least five minutes, foreign material removed, and then rinsed with plain water. Irrigation with an agent that will kill the virus (e.g. 0.01% aqueous iodine, povidone iodine, or even gin or whisky—40 per cent alcohol!) further reduces the risk. The child should be taken to a local medical practitioner as soon as possible (**not wait until return to the UK**) and a specific query made about rabies prophylaxis, as well as a tetanus booster if necessary (parents have confused these two). They need to know that rabies prophylaxis is a course of several injections and that the full course is essential. It consists of human rabies immunoglobulin (HRIG) given as soon as possible (20 iu/kg) half irrigating the wound, half intramuscularly. Then a course of human diploid-cell rabies vaccine is started in 1 ml doses, one immediately and then on days 3, 7, 14, 30, and 90. It is given by deep sc injection (away from the site where HRIG was given). In the immunized individual only three injections are needed, one immediately and then on days 7 and 90. **The course may be stopped if the diagnosis is refuted by the animal surviving.**

Meningitis

Unlicensed meningococcal vaccines are available on a named-patient basis against Groups A and C. Their use is dependent on the current epidemiology of meningococcal infection in the world. Thus in 1987 they were recommended for visitors to the Middle East who were going to be living in crowded conditions, because of an epidemic Group A disease in Saudi Arabia associated with pilgrims attending a religious festival. The same argument would apply for visitors to the meningococcal belt in West Africa who will be visiting rural areas.

European tick-borne encephalitis (TBE)

Austria is the most likely country of exposure but the disease occurs from Scandinavia to the Balkans and from Alsace to Western USSR. Most cases of TBE in these countries occur in June and July with a smaller peak in October. It is a serious disease which can cause death or permanent disability. The virus is spread by the common wood tick and the only risk is to persons who trek through or camp near densely forested areas. Some protection is afforded by using stout footwear and an insect repellant. A safe, highly effective unlicensed killed vaccine is available on a named-patient basis from the manufacturers (see below) and further information on its use can be obtained from a national advice centre. Two doses are recommended, at a four- to six-week interval, the second at least two weeks before possible exposure, with a booster at 12 months and three-yearly if there is a continued risk.

Vaccine is available on a named-patient basis from: Immuno Ltd, Arctic House, Rye Lane, Dunton Green, Sevenoaks, Kent TN41 5HB.
Tel: 0732–458101.

TRAVEL ADVICE AND IMMUNIZATION
CONSULTATION PLAN

This will be modified in practice, depending on the child's immunization and medical history, the interval between first consultation and departure, and the proposed itinerary.

1. Six to eight weeks before departure: obtain details of exact itinerary, lifestyle, and past immunization history. From this, plan immunization required. If appropriate, start with:

BCG (after tuberculin test);
typhoid;
tetanus booster;
arrange/advise yellow fever for 4 weeks' time at nearest centre;
appointment for OPV booster at **same time**.

2. Two to four weeks before departure:

Confirm yellow fever given;
if indicated, administer: measles, OPV, second typhoid, second cholera;
give general advice about hygiene, food, water, rabies.

3. A week before departure: if indicated, immunoglobulin (HNIG).

The child travelling from abroad

The two main groups are families returning from a short stay in Europe or the Mediterranean, and travellers from the Indian subcontinent or Africa (West or East), either after a long stay or as new immigrants.

The child with an infection most commonly presents with fever and/or gastrointestinal symptoms. Some points to consider for any child (or adult) recently returned are:

1. Any fever in such a person or a contact requires urgent investigation. Many travel-acquired infections have implications for contacts and are notifiable. Also, not all imported infections occur clinically in the traveller. The first case may be in a UK contact who has never been abroad. Examples of this have occurred for meningococcal meningitis type A, typhoid, polio, diphtheria, hepatitis A, and non-enteric salmonellosis.

2. Not all imported infections are necessarily exotic: the commonest are gastroenteritis due to *Salmonella*, *Campylobacter*, *Shigella*, and *E. coli*.

3. There should be a higher diagnostic suspicion for diseases which used to be prevalent in UK children, such as diphtheria, polio, and tuberculosis, especially in children of immigrants entering the country for the first time or who may have been away on extended visits and whose immunizations are likely to be less than required.

4. Most new immigrants will be underimmunized (parents as well as children) and catch-up schedules should be used (see p. 311).

Diagnosis and public-health management

The individual coming from abroad could have almost any infectious disease and space precludes detailed reference to all possibilities. The BMA publish a useful guide (see Further reading, no. 12,

p. 332). Benenson's guide (Further reading, no. 2) is also highly recommended, though it only comes into its own once the diagnosis has been made.

Some pointers for action are:

1. Take a country-by-country history with dates (of family contacts if the child has not recently been abroad) and consult a specialist.

2. Malaria must be considered in a child who has been in an endemic zone, however long ago. It may be falciparum, which can kill if not treated early.

3. If malaria can be excluded in a **fever** with non-specific symptoms and/or rash, consider typhoid, hepatitis A, meningococcal infection, or tuberculosis. There is always concern about Lassa fever in returnees from West Africa. However, none of the 10 importations 1971–87 have been in children, although it does occur at young ages in endemic zones. The common bacterial causes of **gastroenteritis** are listed on p. 57. A profuse watery diarrhoea may be due to cholera (not all of which is epidemic— see Table 14). Prolonged diarrhoea and non-specific abdominal symptoms may be caused by *Giardia lamblia*. It is also important to look for some of the intestinal worms, both exotic and commonplace. This can be done by a stool specimen, requesting microscopy and detailing the country of origin.

4. If there is **fever and sore throat**, consider diphtheria, and look for weeping skin lesions among close contacts, which may be cutaneous diphtheria. If **fever is combined with neurological symptoms**, typhoid, malaria and meningitis may present this way; also consider rabies. Poliomyelitis may be the cause of aseptic meningitis or a febrile illness with paralysis in a recent returnee. With **fever and jaundice** the commonest causes are viral hepatitis and falciparum malaria. A rare possibility in a very sick patient is yellow fever.

Post-holiday rabies concerns

Increasing public awareness of rabies and foreign travel has led to increasing demand for advice about possible exposure. The following history should be taken:

1. Personal. Name, age, sex, weight, address of the child, and family telephone number.

2. The exposure. Type (bite/lick/scratch, etc.). Where on the body? Was the skin broken? (Examine the site.) When did it occur and what was the exact geographic location? Details of local advice or management of the wound, including name, site, and number of vaccinations given.

3. The animal. Species, wild or domestic? Name, telephone number, and address of owners known? Was the animal provoked (e.g. child teasing it), and was it behaving oddly? Did it look ill? What happened to it subsequently? **If the animal was known to be alive 14 days after the bite, rabies can be excluded**.

4. Were local public health authorities informed? Was the animal's brain being examined? If so, appropriate names, addresses, and telephone numbers.

There will be some circumstances, e.g. dog-bite in India, where the high risk will be clear and post-exposure prophylaxis with human rabies immunoglobulin (HRIG) (half around wound, half intra-muscular) and HDCRV (into upper arm, not buttock) must be started immediately. Sources of vaccine and HRIG are given on p. 000 and these centres should also be consulted about any suspected cases. If in doubt, ask! A delay of weeks or even months after an exposure is **not** a contraindication to prophylaxis. Domestic animals can often be traced through local British Embassies via DHSS International Division (consult DHSS direct (01–470 1255) or the CDSC (01–200 6868) may advise.

A short list of the actions to be taken for these important diseases is shown in Table 15.

Table 15 Major health actions needed for principal serious imported diseases in the UK

Infection	Notifiable	Public-health measures in UK	Reference
Typhoid and paratyphoid	Yes*	Case should be admitted to infectious disease unit (IDU)	PHLS salmonella subcommittee: Notes on the control of human sources of gastrointestinal infections, infestations, and bacterial intoxications in the UK available from PHLS CDSC
		Screen household contacts. Exclusion from nursery/infant school until 3 negative stool and urine specimens at weekly intervals beginning after clinical recovery; hygiene education.	
Cholera	Yes* but only if *V. cholerae* 01 isolated (often non-cholera vibrios can cause watery diarrhoea)	Case admitted to IDU. Clinical surveillance of household contacts for 5 days after last exposure to case or source; hygiene education. NB: no risk epidemic cholera in UK these days	
Malaria	Yes	None	—
Yellow fever	Yes	None	—
Rabies	Yes*	Patient admitted to high-security unit. Close contacts offered post-exposure vaccination	DHSS memorandum on Rabies, 1977. London: HMSO
Viral haemorrhagic fever (Lassa, Marburg, Ebola)	Yes*	Patient admitted to high-security unit. Clinical surveillance of close contacts	DHSS memorandum on the control of viral haemorrhagic fevers, 1986. London: HMSO

* For all suspected or confirmed cases also inform CDSC by telephone: 01–200 6868 (24 hours and weekends), ask for duty doctor.

Appendices

Appendix 1

NOTIFIABLE DISEASES (as October 1 1988)

	England and Wales	Northern Ireland	Scotland
Acute encephalitis	+	+	0
Acute poliomyelitis	+	+	+
Anthrax	+	+	+
Chickenpox	0	0	+
Cholera	+	+	+
Diphtheria	+	+	+
Dysentery (amoebic or bacillary)	+	+	+
Erysipelas	0	0	+
Food poisoning (all sources)	+	+	+
Legionella	0	0	+
Leprosy	+	0	+
Leptospirosis	+	0	Leptospiral jaundice
Malaria	+	0	+
Measles	+	+	+
Membranous croup	0	0	+
Meningitis	+	+	0
Meningococcal septicaemia (without meningitis)	+	+	+
Mumps	+	+	+
Ophthalmia neonatorum,			

	Medical Officer of Environmental Health of the local authority (or officer performing his function)	Chief Administrative Medical Officer of the appropriate Health and Social Services Board	Chief Administrative Medical Officer of the appropriate Health Board
trachomatis infection	+	0	+
Paratyphoid fever	+	+	+
Plague	+	+	+
Puerperal fever	0	0	+
Rabies	+	+	+
Relapsing fever	+	+	+
Rubella	+	+	+
Scarlet fever	+	+	+
Smallpox	+	+	+
Tetanus	+	0	0
Tuberculosis	+	+	+
Typhoid fever	+	+	+
Typhus	+	+	+
Viral haemorrhagic fever	+	+	+
Viral hepatitis	+	+	+
Whooping cough	+	+	+
Yellow fever	+	+	+
Notify	Medical Officer of Environmental Health of the local authority (or officer performing his function)	Chief Administrative Medical Officer of the appropriate Health and Social Services Board	Chief Administrative Medical Officer of the appropriate Health Board

Report AIDS cases on a special AIDS Clinical Report Form in strict medical confidence to the Director, PHLS CDSC, 61 Colinsdale Avenue, London NW9 5EQ.

Appendix 2
ANTI-MICROBIALS

Drug	Route	Times Daily	Usual individual dosage					Comments
			Birth*	1 year	7 years	14 years		
Acyclovir	iv	3	15 mg/kg					Zovirax: used for severe neonatal HSV infection, herpes encephalitis, eczema herpeticum, and varicella in immunocompromized children
Amikacin	im iv	2	7.5 mg/kg	100 mg	200 mg	500 mg		Amikin: aminoglycoside sometimes used for severe Gram-negative infections, i.e. cystic fibrosis Check renal function prior to use
Amoxycillin	o im iv	3	31 mg	62.5 mg	125 mg	250 mg		Amoxil: treatment of otitis media, pneumonia, etc; standard course 5 days

For severe infections such as meningitis use 200 mg/kg/day (100 mg/kg/day for neonates) iv, 6 hourly for 10 days
For im use mix with 1% lignocaine instead of water

Amoxycillin and clavulanic acid	o iv	3	31 mg	62.5 mg	125 mg	250 mg

Augmentin: clavulanic acid is beta-lactamase inhibitor; broadens spectrum of amoxycillin to include most *Staphylococcus aureus* penicillinase-producing strains

Amphotericin	iv (infuse over 6 hours)	1	250 microgram/kg

Fungizone: fungal, esp. candidal septicaemia, usually in neonate or immunocompromized child
Increase dose gradually over several days to 1 mg/kg
Several weeks therapy may be required
Watch renal tubular function

Drug	Route	Times Daily	Usual individual dosage				Comments
			Birth*	1 year	7 years	14 years	
Ampicillin	o im iv	4	62.5 mg tds	125 mg	250 mg	500 mg	Penbritin: otitis media, pneumonia, and meningitis Standard course 5 days For major infections, i.e. meningitis, use 400 mg/kg/day (200 mg/kg/day neonates) 4 hourly for 7–10 days
Azlocillin	iv	3	100 mg/kg (bd)	750 mg	2 g	3 g	Securopen: treatment of pseudomonas septicaemia (immunocompromized child) and cystic fibrosis Contraindicated in penicillin allergy
Benzylpenicillin	See penicillin G						
Carbenicillin	iv	4	50 mg/kg	100 mg/kg	100 mg/kg	100 mg/kg	Pyopen: used to treat pseudomonas infections in immunocompromized child...

Drug	Route	Doses	Dose (<1 wk)	Dose	High dose	Notes
						load—1 gram contains 5.4 mmol Na$^+$ Being superseded by newer penicillins and aminoglycosides
Cefotaxime	iv	3	65 mg/kg (<1 wk 100 mg/kg twice daily)	33–66 mg/kg	500 mg–1 g	Claforan: treatment of septicaemia, neonatal meningitis, and life-threatening infections, esp. if pseudomonas infection suspected Reduce dose in renal failure Max. doses in meningitis
Ceftazidime	iv im	3	12 5–30 mg (bd)	10–30 mg/kg High dosage 50 mg/kg		Fortum: broad spectrum Particularly effective in *Pseudomonas aeruginosa* infections Use high dose in children with cystic fibrosis, meningitis, and the immunocompromized
Cefuroxime	iv	3	20–40 mg/kg (< 1 wk bd)	20–40 mg/kg	375–750 mg 750 mg– 1.5 g	Zinacef: *H. influenzae* infections and neonatal sepsis Reduce dose in renal impairment Use max. dose in meningitis

Drug	Route	Times Daily	Usual individual dosage				Comments
			Birth*	1 year	7 years	14 years	
Cephradine	o iv im	4	—	125–250 mg	250–500 mg	500 mg–1 g	Velosef: treatment of infections, i.e. orthopaedic and urine infections if resistant organisms Reduce dose in renal impairment
Chloramphenicol	o iv	4	(< 1 wk od > 1 wk bd)	25 mg/kg	—	—	Chloromycetin: only used for treatment of meningitis, epiglottitis, and some cases of typhoid Monitor levels in neonates and in children having concurrent phenobarbitone High dose ampicillin/penicillin G can be substituted if organism sensitive to these drugs Well absorbed orally

Drug	Route					Notes
Chloroquine	o				Initially 10 mg/kg to a maximum of 600 mg; 6 hours later 5 mg/kg; then 5 mg/kg per day, daily dose for 2 days	For initial treatment of simple malaria when chloroquine resistance is not a problem
Clotrimazole	o	3			Use topically	Fungal infection—*Tinea pedis* (athlete's foot)
Co-trimoxazole	o iv (infusion 1½ h)	2	—	240 mg	480 mg 960 mg	Bactrim/Septrin: urinary tract infections, chest infections, typhoid, invasive salmonellosis. Drug is mixture of 5 parts sulphamethoxazole and 1 part trimethoprim (dose = sum of each in mg). For urine infection prophylaxis use once daily. In Pneumocystis pneumonia 120 mg/kg/day given 6 hourly
Diethylcarbamazine	o			—	9–12 mg/kg	Banocide: discuss treatment with specialist

Drug	Route	Times Daily	Usual individual dosage				Comments
			Birth*	1 year	7 years	14 years	
Erythromycin	o	4	< 1 wk 10 mg/kg > 1 wk bd > 1 wk tds 12 mg/kg	125 mg	250 mg	500 mg	Erythroped: use when definite history of penicillin allergy
	iv continuous (infusion)		12 mg/kg	12 mg/kg			Treatment of *Chlamydia trachomatis*, *C. psittaci*, and *Legionella* infections
Ethambutol	o	1	—	—	25 mg/kg		Myambutol: treatment of tuberculosis
							Used in conjunction with isoniazid and/or rifampicin
							Avoid in renal impairment
							Visual problems can result and it should not be given to children < 6 yr
							Reduce dose after 60 days to 15 mg/kg/day if still required

Drug	Route	Freq/day	Neonate			Adult	Comments
Flucloxacillin	o iv im	4 (0–2 wk bd)	62.5 mg	125 mg	250 mg	500 mg	Floxapen: staphylococcal infections—septicaemia and osteomyelitis May be combined with another antibiotic Drain any abscess surgically In life-threatening situations use 200 mg/kg/day given 6 hourly iv
Fusidic acid	o iv	3 3	50 mg/kg 62.5 mg	250 mg 125 mg	500 mg 250 mg	750 mg 500 mg	Fucidin: osteomyelitis and suppurative arthritis May be combined with flucloxacillin or erythromycin Oral dose expressed as fusidic acid, iv dose as sodium fusidate
Gentamicin	iv im	3	2 mg/kg < 1 wk 2 mg/kg bd > 1 wk 3 mg/kg bd	2 mg/kg	2 mg/kg		Genticin: Gram-negative infections, neonatal sepsis, cystic fibrosis Always monitor trough and peak levels Children with cystic fibrosis may need higher doses

Drug	Route	Times Daily	Usual individual dosage				Comments
			Birth*	1 year	7 years	14 years	
Griseofulvin	o	2	—		5 mg/kg		For ringworm of scalp (6 weeks), nails (6 months) May cause photosensitivity
Isoniazid	o im iv	1	3–10 mg/kg	10 mg/kg	200 mg	300 mg	Treatment of tuberculosis Combined with other drugs unless for prophylaxis **For TB meningitis** use 10–20 mg/kg
Mebendazole	o	1	—	—	100 mg if 2 yrs and older		Vermox Contraindicated in children under 2 years of age
Metronidazole	o pr iv (20 min) o	3 3 3 1	— — —	7.5 mg/kg 250 mg 7.5 mg/kg 500 mg	500 mg 800 mg	1 g 2 g	Flagyl: treatment and prophylaxis of anaerobic infections, esp. appendicitis, giardiasis, amoebiasis Full treatment doses for anaerobic infections shown with 3-times-daily regimens; rrear for 5–7 days

Drug	Route	No.					Notes
Miconazole	o iv (30 min)	4 3	62.5 mg	62.5 mg 12–15 mg/kg	125 mg	125–250 mg	Daktarin: fungal infections esp. *Candida* Oral preparation for oral thrush Discuss with microbiologist before using for systemic candidiasis
Netilmicin	iv im	3	2 mg/kg < 1 wk 2 mg/kg/bd > 1 wk 3 mg/kg/bd		2 mg/kg		Netillin: Gram-negative infections Neonatal sepsis, cystic fibrosis Always monitor levels Children with cystic fibrosis often need higher dosage
Nitrofurantoin	o	4	Avoid in neonatal period		100 mg		For urinary-tract infections with multiple organism resistance May cause nausea and vomiting
Nystatin	o or topical 3 or 4						Given for oral thrush or infantile eczema infected with *Candida*

Drug	Route	Times Daily	Usual individual dosage					Comments
			Birth*	1 year	7 years	14 years		
Penicillin G (benzylpenicillin)	im	4	50 mg	150 mg	300 mg	600 mg		Crystapen: 1 megaunit = 600 mg
	iv	6	< 1 wk 15–30 mg/kg tds > 1 wk 20–45 mg/kg qds	150–500 mg	300–1200 mg	600–2400 mg		Tonsillitis, lobar pneumonia, erysipelas, endocarditis, meningococcal, and pneumococcal meningitis Always use max. dose iv in infective endocarditis or meningitis
Penicillin G as procaine penicillin	im	1	60 mg/kg to maximum of 2.4 g					For treatment of gonococcal infection in childhood Therapeutic level maintained better with Probenecid given 30 minutes before injection (1 gm, oral)
Penicillin V (phenoxymethyl-penicillin)	o	4	62.5 mg	125 mg	250 mg	500 mg		Tonsillitis and minor infections, prophylaxis of rheumatic fever and septicaemia after splenectomy

Drug	Route	No. of doses	Dose (<1 y)				Notes
Piperacillin	iv	2–4	50–100 mg (bd) or tds			50–100 mg/kg	Pneumonia after initial iv/im penicillin. Prophylactic usage can be given once or twice daily in doses shown. Pipril: for treatment of *Pseudomonas aeruginosa* infection in children with cystic fibrosis. Combine with aminoglycoside
Piperazine	o	Single doses given 14 days apart (×2)	<1 y 5 ml	10 ml	15 ml	15 ml	Dose as for Pripsen sachet (4 g piperazine sulphate and 15.3 mg sennosides per sachet of 1.5 ml)
Pivampicillin	o	3	175 mg	175 mg	175 mg	250 mg	Pondocillin: 175 mg in 5 ml. Similar antibacterial spectrum as ampicillin, with better absorption
Pyrazinamide	o	1	—			20–30 mg/kg	Zinamide: used in tuberculous meningitis. Not licensed for use in children in UK (see p. 143). Watch liver function

Drug	Route	Times Daily	Usual individual dosage				Comments
			Birth*	1 year	7 years	14 years	
Quinine	o	3	60 mg	125 mg	300 mg	600 mg	Doses given as base
	iv (over 4 h)	3		10 mg/kg			Quinine base, 100 mg = quinine bisulphate 169 mg = quinine dihydrochloride/hydrochloride or quinine sulphate 122 mg
							Treatment of malaria, esp. if chloroquine resistance, or cerebral malaria
							With resistant strains an iv loading dose of 20 mg/kg is required, switch to oral therapy as soon as possible
							Always seek specialist advice
							Treatment usually given for 10–14 days
							iv therapy only given > 3 months, oral from birth

Drug	Route	Frequency (per day)	Dose	Dose	Dose	Notes
			10 mg/kg	20 mg/kg	(maximum dosage 600 mg) 600 mg 600 mg	Rifadin: treatment of tuberculosis
(as prophylaxis)	iv	2 (for 2 days) 2 (for 4 days)	10 mg/kg	10 mg/kg	(maximum dosage 600 mg)	Prophylaxis of *Neisseria meningitidis* infection
	o			10 mg/kg		Prophylaxis of *Haemophilus influenzae* infection
						Warn about orange secretions
						Drug interaction with oral contraceptive
Streptomycin	im	1	—	30–40 mg/kg	30–40 1 g mg/kg	Treatment of tuberculous meningitis for first few weeks (not more than 12)
						Other antituberculous drugs also always given simultaneously
Thiabendazole	o	2			25 mg/kg	Mintezol: treatment of refractory hookworm, threadworm, whipworm, roundworm, visceral larva migrans, *Strongyloides*
						Treatment given for 2–7 days—see literature

Drug	Route	Times Daily	Usual individual dosage				Comments
			Birth*	1 year	7 years	14 years	
Trimethoprim	o	2	50 mg avoid in neonatal period	50 mg	100 mg 3–4.5 mg/kg	200 mg	For urinary-tract infections
	iv	2					Single evening dose as prophylaxis

*Special care should be taken in prescribing antibiotics in the neonatal period, particularly for preterm infants and specialist texts should be consulted in this situation, as the dosages given may not be appropriate in all circumstances.
Key: bd = twice daily; tds = three times daily; qds = four times daily.

Appendix 3

RAPID GUIDE TO EXCLUSION PERIODS

(See also main text. Note: includes some illnesses not described in text.)

Disease	Incubation period (time from meeting organisms to first symptoms)	
	Common range	Extreme range
Amoebic dysentery*	Variable, commonly 2–4 weeks	
Campylobacter gastroenteritis	3–5 days	1–10 days
Chickenpox	13–17 days	13–21 days
Cholera*	2–3 days	few hours to 5 days
Diphtheria*	2–5 days	2–7 days
E. coli	1–6 days	
Fifth disease	5–22 days	
Gastroenteritis: *Campylobacter*/rotavirus/*Shigella*/typhoid—see individual notes		
Giardiasis	Variable 5–25 days	—

Infectious period (when child may pass on disease)	Type of spread and infectivity (how easily child can pass on the disease)	Exclusion period
May be prolonged	Food/water, faecal hand–mouth Inf: Moderate	(MOEH) Until 3 stool specimens negative for cysts
Infectious throughout illness—until antibiotic given	Food/water faecal hand mouth Inf: Moderate	Until asymptomatic
1–2 days before rash appears to 6 days after rash first appears	Nearby persons—droplet or contact Inf: High	Until 6 days from appearance of rash
Variable—until stools are negative	Contaminated food or water Inf: High	(MOEH)
Variable; usually 2–4 weeks from first signs There are carriers	Nearby persons—contact Inf: Moderate	(MOEH)
Variable; may be prolonged beyond diarrhoea	Faecal hand–mouth Inf: Moderate	(MOEH)
Unknown	Unclear	None
During symptoms There are carriers	Faecal hand–mouth Inf: Low	None

Disease	Incubation period (time from meeting organisms to first symptoms)	
	Common range	Extreme range
Glandular fever	4–6 weeks	—
Hand, foot, and mouth disease (Coxsackie virus)	3–5 days	—
Hepatitis A* (infectious hepatitis)	28–30 days	15–50 days
Hepatitis B* (serum H)	60–90 days	45–160 days
Herpes simplex (cold sores)	2–12 days	—
Impetigo—streptococcal/ staphylococcal	1–3 days 4–10 days	— —
Influenza	2–3 days	—
Malaria*	12–30 days	8–10 months from one rare type
Measles*	8–13 days to fever 10–15 days to rash	—
Meningococcal disease*	3–4 days	2–10 days
Molluscum contagiosum	2–7 weeks	—

...fectious period (when child may ...ass on disease)	Type of spread and infectivity (how easily child can pass on the disease)	Exclusion period
...rolonged beyond illness ...here are carriers	Very close contact Inf: Low	Nil for schoolchildren
...cute phase of illness	Nearby persons—contact, faecal hand-mouth and droplet Inf: Low	During acute phase of illness
...4 days before jaundice to 7 days after	Contact by hand, faecal oral, and contaminated food or water Inf: Moderate	7 days from jaundice starting
...nfectious before and after illness ...here are carriers	Very close contact or contaminated blood Inf: Very low	Nil once well
...ariable	Close contact Inf: Moderate	Nil
...hile lesions are draining	By contact Inf: High	Until lesions have healed
...he 3 days before onset of symptoms	Nearby persons by droplet Inf: High	Nil once well
—	Not infectious in UK	Nil
...rom first symptoms until 4 days after rash appears ...ow risk after 2 days of rash	Nearby persons—droplet Inf: Very high	Until 4 days after appearance of rash
...here are carriers	Nearby persons—droplet Inf: Moderate	Seek advice (MOEH)
...s long as lesions persist	Very close contact Inf: Very low	Nil

Disease	Incubation period (time from meeting organisms to first symptoms)	
	Common range	Extreme range
Mumps*	18 days	14–21 days
Nits/head lice (*Pediculosis capitis*)	7 days	—
Polio*	7–14 days	3–35 days
Ringworm (scalp	10–14 days	—
Ringworm (body)	4–10 days	—
Ringworm (feet) (athletes' foot)	Unknown	—
Rotavirus	48 h approx.	—
Rubella* **	16–18 days	14–23 days
Scabies	days to weeks	—
Shigella* (bacillary dysentery)	1–3 days	1–7 days
Tetanus*	4–10 days	4–21 days
Tuberculosis*	4–12 weeks	—
Typhoid*	1–3 weeks	—

nfectious period (when child may pass on disease)	Type of spread and infectivity (how easily child can pass on the disease)	Exclusion period
days before swelling to 9 days after Max. 2 days before swelling	Nearby contact—droplet Inf: High	For 7 days after swelling has appeared
As long as lice remain alive or hair is untreated	Very close contact Inf: Low	Until all lice dead and hair treated
Via faeces for 3–6 weeks	Nearby—faeces, hand, mouth Inf: High	Seek advice (MOEH)
As long as lesions are present	All by direct contact Inf: Low	Until lesions are healing esp. in younger children in day care (NB: not feet ringworm)
Usually until 8th day of illness	Faecal hand mouth Inf: Moderate	Until diarrhoea ceases
days before rash until 4 days after	Nearby—droplet or contact Inf: High	Until 4 days after rash appears
Until mites and eggs destroyed by two treatments	Very close contact Inf: Low	Until after treatment has started
Usually while symptomatic and in the carrier state	Faecal, hand–mouth Inf: High	Until 3 stool specimens negative (MOEH)
No person-to-person spread	From soil Inf: Nil	Nil
Variable	By close contact Inf: Low	(MOEH and chest physician)
Until stool clear	Faecal hand–mouth Inf: Moderate	Until 3 stools negative

Disease	Incubation period (time from meeting organisms to first symptoms)	
	Common range	Extreme range
Warts and verrucae	4 months	1–12 months
Whooping cough*	7–10 days	7–21 days

*   Notifiable disease.
**   see congenital rubella (p. 118) *re* notification.
MOEH   Consultation with Medical Officer of Environmental Health (or alter
Note: Information on gastrointestinal infection derived from Communicable I

Infectious period (when child may pass on disease)	Type of spread and infectivity (how easily child can pass on the disease)	Exclusion period
Unknown, possibly as long as lesion lasts	Very close contact Inf: V. low	Nil
Up to 3 weeks after paroxysmal coughing starts or until 7 days after antibiotic commences	Droplet Inf: High	5 days from starting antibiotic treatment

er) advised.
ort, Supplement 1, 1983 (see Further reading, Appendix 7).

Appendix 4

Pre-school

Birth	BCG for babies in Asian and other immigrant families with high TB rates and those in contact with active respiratory tuberculosis
3 months	Polio + diphtheria/tetanus/pertussis (DTP)
4.5–5 months (i.e. 6–8 weeks after first injection)	Polio + DTP
8.5–11 months (i.e. 4–6 months after second injection)	Polio + DTP
12–24 months (preferably at 15 months to ensure early and lasting immunity)	Combined measles, mumps, and rubella (MMR) or measles

Note: In children over 3, the three injections of DTP and polio drops can be given at monthly intervals.

Pre-school

4–5 years	MMR, if not previously given, + polio + diphtheria/tetanus booster

Secondary school

10–14 years	Heaf or Mantoux and, if negative, BCG
10–14 years	Rubella (girls only)

School leaving

15–19 years Polio + Tetanus

Accelerated schedule

Only recommended if rapid protection needed (e.g. during pertussis epidemic)

3 months Polio + Triple
4 months Polio + Triple
5 months Polio + Triple
15 months MMR or measles **plus** additional Triple and polio

Schedules for unimmunized children

(Primary schedule for an unimmunized child (subject to the usual contraindications)

Under 3 First injection MMR (or
    measles) + diphtheria/tetanus/pertussis
    (DTP) + polio
    After 2 months DTP + polio
    After another 5 months DTP + polio
    Booster after 3 years

Age 3–6th First injection MMR or (measles) + DTP + polio
birthday After 1 month DTP + polio
    After another month DTP + polio
    Booster after 3 years

Age 6–10th First injection MMR (or measles) + DTP* or
 birthday Dip/Tet* + polio
    After 1 month DTP* or Dip/Tet* + polio
    After another month DTP* or Dip/Tet* + polio
    Booster after 3 years

Over 10 Consider Heaf/Mantoux (Asian child)
    First injection MMR (or measles) + low-dose
    diphtheria** (see p. 000) + tetanus + polio
    After 1 month low-dose diphtheria + tetanus + polio
    After another month low-dose
    diphtheria + tetanus + polio

Girls over 14 also need a rubella injection if they have not had one.

*Where young siblings are at risk of catching whooping cough older children should be offered DTP not diphtheria/tetanus.

Note: Three years should elapse between giving the primary course and the pre-school booster of diphtheria/tetanus and polio.

**This requires three injections at the first visit, which is asking a lot of the child's and the parents' stamina. It may be best to leave out diphtheria on the first occasion and give a third dose one month after stage 3.

Schedules for catching up with whooping cough

Schedule for catching up with whooping cough, e.g. where parents have decided they want their child to have the injection having missed out beforehand.

Under 3 years	First injection pertussis (monovalent)
	After 2 months pertussis
	After another 2 months pertussis
After 3rd birthday	First injection pertussis
	After 1 month pertussis
	After another month pertussis

If other first-year injections need catching up they can also be given at monthly intervals once a child is over 3.

Appendix 5

Public Health Laboratories

Note: all of these hold post-exposure courses for rabies prophylaxis.

England and Wales

Central PHLS, Communicable Disease Surveillance Centre, Tel.: 01–200 6868.
PHLS Virus Reference Laboratory, Tel.: 01–200 4400

PHL Ashford	0233 35731
PHL Bath	0225 28331
PHL Birmingham	021–772 4311
PHL Brighton	0273 603506
PHL Cambridge	0223 242111
PHL Cardiff	0222 755944
PHL Dorchester	0305 64478
PHL Epsom	03727 26633
PHL Exeter	0392 77833
PHL Gloucester	0452 35334
PHL Guildford	0483 66091
PHL Leeds	0532 645011
PHL Liverpool	051–525 2323
PHL Luton	0582 53211
PHL Newcastle	0632 738811
PHL Norwich	0603 611816
PHL Nottingham	0602 421421
PHL Oxford	0865 60631
PHL Poole	0202 675771
PHL Portsmouth	0705 822331
PHL Sheffield	0742 387749
PHL Taunton	0823 8557/8
PHL Watford	0923 44366

Scotland

Doctors should contact local laboratories, Health Board Communicable Disease Centre Departments, or the Communicable Disease (Scotland) Unit, Tel.: 041–946 7120.

Information centres for travel

These prefer telephone consultations from the patient's doctor.

England

International Relations,
(Health) Branch, DHSS,
Alexander Fleming House,
Elephant and Castle,
London SE1 6BY.
Tel.: 01–407 5522, Ext. 6749, 6711

Public Health Laboratory Service,
Communicable Disease Surveillance Centre,
61 Colindale Avenue,
London NW9 5EQ.
Tel.: 01–200 6868 (ask for duty doctor)

Wales

Welsh Office,
Cathays Park,
Cardiff CF1 3NQ.
Tel.: 0222 82511, Ext. 3336

Scotland

Scottish Home and Health Dept,
St. Andrew's House,
Edinburgh EH1 3DE.
Tel.: 031–556 8501, Ext. 2438

For vaccination information, hard advice, and post-exposure course for rabies prophylaxis:

The Communicable Disease (Scotland) Unit,
Ruchill Hospital,
Bilsland Drive,
Glasgow G20 9NB.
Tel.: 041–946 7120

Northern Ireland

DHSS, Dundonald House,
Upper Newtownards Road,
Belfast BT4 3SF.
Tel.: 0232 63939, Ext. 2593

For post-exposure rabies prophylaxis course and advice, Tel.: 0232 65011,
Ext. 758.

Other centres

Malaria Reference Laboratory,
London School of Hygiene and Tropical Medicine,
Keppel Street,
London WC1E 7HT.
Tel · 01–636 7921

Medical Advisory Reference for Travellers Abroad (MASTA),
Bureau of Hygiene and Tropical Diseases,
Keppel Street,
London WC1E 7HT.
Tel.: 01–636 8636

British Airways Medical Centre,
75 Regent Street,
London W1.
Tel.: 01–439 9584

Provides advice to public and profession immunization service (all vaccines
available).

Appendix 6

SOURCES OF SUPPLY OF VACCINES AND OTHER IMMUNOLOGICAL PRODUCTS

In compiling this list, the Department of Health and Social Security adopted the following practice:

1. a. Where a blood product is available from the Blood Products Laboratory (BPL), this is the only source listed. Alternative commercial suppliers of licensed products, although they may exist, are not included.

   b. Where a UK product licence has been granted, no unlicensed sources of supply are shown.

   Products listed as having no known source have been included for several reasons:

   i. Enquiries have been received by the Department as to their availability.

   ii. The product was formerly available.

   iii. The product has been mentioned in medical literature.

2. The list is not comprehensive and the inclusion or exclusion of a particular product should not be taken to imply that it is either recommended or not recommended for use. Nor does inclusion of unlicensed products imply any warranty as to their safety or efficacy.

3. A number of items listed are not covered by product licences under the Medicines Act 1968, and are available only on a 'named patient' basis, (Section 9(1) and 13(1) of the Medicines Act 1968). For such items the detailed statutory conditions applicable are set out in SI 673/1984. It should be noted that any practitioner prescribing an unlicensed product does so entirely on his own responsibility and carries the total burden for the patient's welfare. Guidance notes on the provisions affecting Doctors and Dentists are available in Medicines Act Leaflet (MAL) 30, available from the DHSS, Market Towers, 1 Nine Elms Lane, London SW8 5NQ.

4. *DISCLAIMER.* The Department of Health and Social Security accepts no responsibility for, and disclaims liability in respect of any vaccines or immunological products in this list and medical practitioners who prescribe them for patients do so entirely on their own responsibility and upon their own clinical judgement.

1. Sources of supply of vaccines and other immunological products

Product	Source of supply
Anthrax vaccine	DHSS Central Contract (see Section 2)
Anti D immunoglobulin	Blood Products Laboratory (BPL) via Regional Transfusion Centres
Antilymphocyte immunoglobulin (equine)	Hoechst, UK
Antilymphocyte Immunoglobulin (rabbit) (N)	Merieux UK Ltd
BCG vaccine (intradermal)	DHSS Central Contract (see Section 2)
BCG vaccine (isoniazid resistant)	Evans Medical Ltd
BCG vaccine (percutaneous)	Evans Medical Ltd
Black Widow Spider antivenin (N)	Merck, Sharp, and Dohme, USA
Blastomycin	No known source
Botulinum antitoxin	See Botulism antitoxin
Botulism antitoxin	DHSS Central Contract (see Section 2)
British Adder antivenin	Regent Laboratories Ltd (see Section 2)
Cholera vaccine	Wellcome
Coccidioidin (N)	Cutter Biologicals, USA
Corynebacterium parvum	Calmic Medical Division
Dick test and control	No known source
Diphtheria antitoxin	Regent Laboratories Ltd
Diphtheria immunoglobulin (N)	Swiss Serum and Vaccine Institute*
Diphtheria vaccine, adsorbed	Wellcome
Diphtheria vaccine for adults	Regent Laboratories Ltd

Product	Source of supply
Diphtheria vaccine TAF	No known source (discontinued)
Diphtheria and tetanus vaccine (plain)	Wellcome
Diphtheria and tetanus vaccine, adsorbed	Wellcome Evans Medical Ltd
Diphtheria, tetanus, and pertussis vaccine (plain)	Wellcome
Diphtheria, tetanus, and pertussis vaccine (adsorbed)	Wellcome
Gas gangrene antitoxin (mixed)	Merieux UK Ltd
Haemophilus influenza type B vaccine (N)	Mead Johnson, USA
Hepatitis B immunoglobulin	BPL, via Central Public Health Laboratory (CPHL)
Hepatitis B vaccine	Thomas Morson Pharmaceuticals Smith Kline and French Ltd
Histoplasmin	No known source
Human normal immunoglobulin	BPL, via Central Public Health Laboratory (CPHL)
Human Normal Immunoglobulin for use with Measles vaccine	BPL, Elstree (Regional Health Authorities hold stocks)
Influenza vaccine, inactivated	Evans Medical Ltd Duphar Laboratories Ltd Merieux UK Ltd
Japanese encephalitis vaccine (N)	Cambridge Self Care Diagnostics Ltd
Kveim antigen	PHLS (CAMR)
Lymphogranuloma venereum antigen	No known source
Measles immunoglobulin (N)	Immuno Ltd
Measles vaccine, live	Evans Medical Ltd Thomas Morson Pharmaceuticals Smith, Kline, and French Ltd

Product	Source of supply
†Measles, mumps, and rubella vaccine (N)	Thomas Morson Pharmaceuticals†
Meningococcal polysaccharide vaccine, group A (N)	Connaught Merieux UK Ltd Smith, Kline, and French Ltd
Meningococcal polysaccharide vaccine, group C (N)	Connaught
Meningococcal polysaccharide vaccine, groups A&C (N)	Connaught Merieux UK Ltd Smith, Kline, and French Ltd
Meningococcal polysaccharide vaccine, groups A, C, Y, and W135 combined (N)	Connaught Smith, Kline, and French Ltd
Mumps immunoglobulin	BPL, via Central Public Health Laboratory (CPHL)
Mumps skin test antigen (N)	Connaught
Mumps vaccine, live	Thomas Morson Pharmaceuticals
Mycobacteria antigens	See Tuberculin PPD, (atypical)
Pertussis vaccine, (plain)	Wellcome
Pertussis vaccine, adsorbed	No known source
Plague vaccine (N)	Cutter Labs Ltd (UK)
Polio immunoglobulin (N)	Immuno Ltd
Polio vaccine, inactivated	DHSS Central Contract (see Section 2)
Polio vaccine, live (oral)	DHSS Central Contract (see Section 2)
Rabies immunoglobulin	BPL via Central Public Health Laboratory (CPHL)
Rabies vaccine (human diploid cell)	Merieux UK Ltd (see Section 2)
Rocky Mountain Spotted Fever vaccine	Experimental, USA

Product	Source of supply
Rubella immunoglobulin (N)	Immuno Ltd (see also BNF 14.5.1)
Rubella vaccine, live	Smith, Kline, and French Ltd Wellcome Thomas Morson Pharmaceuticals
Scarlet Fever prophylaxis/antitoxin	No known source
Schick test and control	Wellcome
Scorpion venom antiserum (N)	Merieux UK Ltd
Smallpox immunoglobulin	BPL, via Central Public Health Laboratory (CPHL)
Smallpox vaccine	Central Public Health Laboratory (CPHL)
Snake venom antisera	DHSS Central Contract (see Section 2)
Snake venom antisera kits	(see Section 2)
Tetanus immunoglobulin (250 IU in approx 2 ml)	BPL via Regional Transfusion Centres
Tetanus immunoglobulin (250 IU in 1 ml)	Wellcome
Tetanus vaccine	Wellcome
Tetanus vaccine, adsorbed	Wellcome Evans Medical Ltd Merieux UK Ltd
Tetanus and pertussis vaccine	No known source
Tick borne encephalitis immunoglobulin (N)	Immuno Ltd
Tick borne encephalitis vaccine (N)	Immuno Ltd
Toxocara antigen	No known source
Trichinella extract	No known source
Tuberculin, old	No known source

Product	Source of supply
Tuberculin PPD (Heaf and Mantoux 10 TU in 0.1 ml)	DHSS Central Contract (see Section 2)
Tuberculin PPD (other strengths)	Evans Medical Ltd
Tuberculin PPD (atypical) Mycobacterium Avium-Intracellulare Composite Antigen (N)	
Mycobacterium Kansasii (N)	PHLS Mycobacterium Reference Unit
Mycobacterium Marinum (N)	
Mycobacterium Xenopi (N)	
Typhoid vaccine	Wellcome
Typhus vaccine (N)	Swiss Serum and Vaccine Institute*
Varicella zoster immunoglobulin	BPL, via Central Public Health Laboratory (CPHL)
Yellow Fever vaccine, live	Wellcome (see Section 2)

(N) Available only on a 'named patient' basis, under sections 9(1) and 13(1) of the Medicines Act 1968.

* Swiss Serum and Vaccine Institute are not willing to deal directly with individual orders for named patient supply in this country. The products mentioned, however, may be obtainable through a Pharmaceutical Importer.

† Shortly to be more widely available.

2. Products available on central contract and those made available by procurement directorate of the DHSS

The following information on supply arrangements for vaccines and other immunological products applies only to England and Wales. Scotland and Northern Ireland have their own arrangements (see BNF Section 14.4).

Most of the information which follows can be found in Section D, pages 1101–1199 of the Health Service Supply Purchasing Guide (HSSPG), copies of which are held by Regional Supplies Officers and Boards of Governors (London Postgraduate Teaching Hospitals). Full addresses and telephone numbers of the sources quoted below can be found in the HSSPG.

In addition, the Chemist and Druggist Directory has a section on 'Emergency Services', (Prophylactic and Therapeutic Products) which lists designated Holding Centres for some of the products mentioned below.

1.   Anthrax vaccine

Available from designated Holding Centres, as follows: Regional Public Health Laboratories in Leeds, Liverpool and Cardiff; Central Public Health Laboratory, London.

This vaccine should be ordered only when required for use, and not stocked locally.

2.   BCG vaccine, intradermal

Available from District Health Authorities, who order supplies from the DHSS, Russell Square, London, or the Welsh Health Common Services Authority, Cardiff.

3.   Botulism antitoxin, types ABE mixed (previous stock *Botulinum* Antitoxin)

Available from the following Holding Centres:

Northern Region
Cumberland Infirmary, Carlisle (Pathology Laboratory)
Newcastle General Hospital (Pharmacy Department)

Yorkshire Region
Castle Hill Hospital, Cottingham (Pharmacy Department)
Leeds General Infirmary (Pharmacy Department)

Trent Region
Nottingham City Hospital (Pharmacy Department)

East Anglia Region
Regional Transfusion and Immuno-Haematology Centre, Cambridge

North West Thames Region
Edgware General Hospital (Pharmacy Department)
Bedford General Hospital, South Wing (Pharmacy Department)
Virus Reference Laboratory, Central Public Health Laboratory

North East Thames Region
North Middlesex Hospital (Bacteriological Department)

South East Thames Region
Kent and Sussex Hospital, Tunbridge Wells (Pharmacy Department)

South West Thames Region
South London Transfusion Centre, Tooting
Epsom District Hospital (Pharmacy Department)

Wessex Region
Southampton General Hospital (Pharmacy Department)

Oxford Region
Northampton General Hospital (Pathology Department)
Royal Berkshire Hospital, Reading (Pharmacy Department)

South Western Region
Ham Green Hospital, Bristol (Pharmacy Department)
Royal Devon and Exeter Hospital, Exeter (Pharmacy Department)
Plymouth General Hospital (Accident and Emergency Department)
Royal Cornwall Hospital, Truro (Pharmacy Department)

West Midlands Region
Selly Oak Hospital, Birmingham (Pharmacy Department)

Mersey Region
Walton Hospital, Liverpool (Pharmacy Department)

North Western Region
Manchester Royal Infirmary (Pharmacy Department)

Wales
Cardiff Royal Infirmary (Pharmacy Department)
Ysbyty Gwynedd, Bangor (Pharmacy Department)
Withybush Hospital, Haverfordwest (Pharmacy Department)
Maelor General Hospital, Clwyd (Pharmacy Department)
Ysbyty Glan Clwyd, Bodelwyddan, Clwyd (Pharmacy Department)
Singleton Hospital, Swansea (Pharmacy Department)

4. Poliomyelitis vaccine (inactivated)

Available on request from:

a. England: Room 220,
                DHSS PD/AD3,
                14 Russell Square,
                London WC1B 5EP.
                Tel: 01–636 6811 Ext 3236

b. Wales: Welsh Health Common Services Authority (WHCSA),
                  Heron House,
                  35/43 Newport Road,
                  Cardiff CF2 1SB.
                  Tel: 0222 471234 Ext 2068

This vaccine should be ordered one dose at a time and only when required
for use. It should not be stocked locally.

5.   Poliomyelitis vaccine, live (oral)

Available from District Health Authorities, who order supplies from the
DHSS, Russell Square, London, the Welsh Health Common Services
Authority, Cardiff, or the Scottish Health Service Common Services Agency,
Edinburgh.

6.   Rabies vaccine (human diploid cell)

Available in accordance with Health Circular HC(77)29, for pre- and post-
exposure vaccination of persons at special risk of contracting rabies in the
course of their work, from: the Central Public Health Laboratory, London;
Regional Public Health Laboratories in Birmingham, Cardiff, Leeds, Liverpool and Newcastle; the Area Public Health Laboratory, Exeter.

  For use in cases other than the above, it is available from Merieux UK
Ltd.

7.   Snake venom antisera

A. DHSS emergency stocks

The DHSS have arranged for emergency stocks of snake venom antisera to
be available from two Holding Centres:

 i. The National Poisons Information Centre,
    New Cross Hospital,
    Avonley Road,
    London SE14 5ER.
    Tel: 01 407 7600

ii. The Pharmacy Department,
    The Walton Hospital,
    Liverpool L9 1EA.
    Tel: 051 525 3611

Antisera stocked at these Holding Centres cover a range of foreign snakes.
Products held are as follows:

Agkistrodon acutus antivenin
Cobra antivenin (Naja naja)
Coral Snake antivenin (Micrurus mipartitus)
Coral Snake antivenin (Micrurus fulvius)
Crotalidae polyvalent antivenin
Echis carinatus antivenin
European Adder antivenin
Green Pit Viper antivenin (Trimeresurus papeorum)
King Cobra antivenin (Ophiophagus hannah)
Lyophilised Polyvalent antisnake venom
Malayan Pit Viper antivenin
Near and Middle East Snake antivenin
Polyvalent snake antivenin
Polyvalent snakebite serum
Russell's Viper antivenin
Tiger Snake antivenin

Further details on the supply arrangements of snake antivenoms for
treating foreign snake bites are to be found in Health Notice HN(78)13, as
amended by HN(86)9 and the Communicable Disease Report CDR 86/07.
Advice on the management of bites by foreign snakes is available from the
National Poisons Information Centre and may also be obtained from:

i. Dr R D G Theakston
    Liverpool School of Tropical Medicine,
    Pembroke Place,
    Liverpool L3.
    Tel: 051 708 9393

ii. Dr B E Juel-Jenson
    Radcliffe Infirmary,
    Oxford OX2 6HE.
    Tel: 0865 249 891 Ext 4590, 4602 or 4879
    (Out of office hours: 0865 62848)

iii. Dr A Warrell
     Nuffield Department of Clinical Medicine,
     John Radcliffe Hospital,
     Headington,
     Oxford OX3 9DU.
     Tel: 0865 64711 Ext 7491, 7398

B.   Snake venom antisera kits

i.   Snake bite antiserum against all inland viperae, including the British Adder, is available from Regent Laboratories Ltd.

ii.   Snake bite antisera against snakes found in the following areas are available from Hoechst:

> Central and North Africa
> Near and Middle East

8.   Tuberculin PPD

The following are available from the District Health Authorities:

i.   Tuberculin PPD 10 TU in 0.1 ml for Mantoux Test.

ii.   Tuberculin PPD 100 000 TU in 1 ml, for Multiple Puncture Test (Heaf Test).

These are distributed to District Health Authorities who order supplies from the DHSS, Russell Square, London, or the Welsh Health Common Services Authority, Cardiff.

9.   Yellow Fever vaccine

Available only to designated Yellow Fever Vaccination Centres, from Wellcome.

3.   Addresses and telephone numbers of suppliers

Blood Products Laboratory (BPL),
Dagger Lane,
Elstree,
Herts WD6 3BX.
Tel: 01 953 6191

Calmic Medical Division,
The Wellcome Foundation Ltd,
Crewe Hall,
Crewe,
Cheshire CW1 1UB.
Tel: 0270 583151

Central Public Health Laboratory (CPHL),
Colindale Avenue,
London NW9 5HT.
Tel: 01 200 4400

Connaught Laboratories Ltd,
1755 Steeles Avenue West,
Willowdale,
M2R 3T4,
Ontario, Canada.
Tel: (416) 667-2701
Telex: 06-22184

Cutter Biologicals,
Division of Miles Laboratories
    Inc.,
2200 Powell Street,
Emeryville,
CA 94662,
USA.
Tel: (800) 227 2720

Cutter Labs Ltd,
Division of Miles Labs,
Stoke Court,
Stoke Poges,
Slough,
Bucks SL2 4ZY.
Tel: 369 5151 Ext 237

Cambridge Self Care Diagnostics
    Ltd,
The Cambridgeshire Business Park,
Angel Drove,
Ely,
Cambridgeshire CB7 4EE.
Tel: 0353 67564

Evans Medical Ltd,
Foster Avenue,
Woodside Park Estate,
Dunstable,
Beds LU5 5PA.
Tel: 0582 608308

Hoechst UK Ltd,
Pharmaceutical Division,
Hoechst House,
Salisbury Road,
Hounslow,
Middlesex TW4 6JH
Tel: 01 570 7712

Immuno Ltd,
Arctic House,
Rye Lane,
Dunton Green,
Near Sevenoaks,
Kent TN14 5HB.
Tel: 0732 458101

Lister Institute of Preventive Medi-
    cine,
Royal National Orthopaedic Hos-
    pital,
Brockley Hill,
Stanmore,
Middlesex.
Tel: 01–954 6297

Mead Johnson Pharmaceutical
    Division,
2404 W Pennsylvania Street,
Evansville, IN 47721 USA.
Tel: 812 426 6000

Merck, Sharp, and Dohme Ltd,
Hertford Road,
Hoddesdon,
Herts EN11 9BU.
Tel: 0992 467272

Merck, Sharp, and Dohme (USA),
Division of Merck and Co. Inc.,
West Point,
PA 19486,
USA.
Tel: (215) 661 5000

Merieux UK Ltd,
Fulmer Hall,
Hay Lane,
Fulmer,
Slough,
Bucks SL3 6HH.
Tel: 02816 2744/2566

PHLS Centre for Applied Micro-
biology and Research,
Porton Down,
Salisbury,
Wiltshire SP4 0JG.
Tel: 0980 610391, Ext 475

PHLS Mycobacterium Reference
Unit,
University Hospital of Wales,
Heath Park,
Cardiff CF4 4XW.
Tel: Cardiff (0222) 755944, Ext
2049

Regent Laboratories Ltd,
Cunard Road,
London SW10 6PN.
Tel: (Day) 01–965 3637

      (Night) 01–864 3613 (Mr
         Woolfe) or
      01–858 1525 (Mr Richards)

(Emergency) Bliss Chemists,
No 5 Marble Arch,
London W1.
Tel: 01–723 6116

Servier Laboratories Ltd,
Fulmer Hall,
Windmill Road,
Fulmer,
Slough,
Bucks SL3 6HH.
Tel: 02816 2744

Smith, Kline, and French Labora-
tories Ltd, Welwyn Garden
City,
Herts AL7 1EY,
Tel: 0707 325111

Thomas Morson Pharmaceuticals
(See Merck Sharp and Dohme Ltd)

Vestric Ltd,
Stonefield Way,
South Ruislip,
Middx.
Tel: 01–845 2323

Wellcome Foundation Ltd,
Crewe Hall,
Crewe,
Cheshire CW1 1UB.
Tel: 0270 583151

Appendix 7

Infectious diseases

1. Krugman, S., Katz, S. L., Gershon, A. A. and Wilfert, C. M. (1985). *Infectious diseases of children.* CV Mosby, St. Louis.
   American, highly detailed tome.
2. Benenson, A. S. (1985). *Control of communicable diseases in man,* (14th edn). American Public Health Association, Washington.
   An excellent practical handbook.
3. Farrar, W. E. and Lambert, H. P. (1984). *Infectious diseases.* Gower, London.
   A short pictorial guide including most of the common rashes.
4. Emond, R. T. D. and Rowland, H. A. K. (1987). *Colour atlas of infectious diseases,* (2nd edn). Wolfe Medical Atlas.
   A more complete pictorial guide.
5. Public Health Laboratory Service Communicable Disease Surveillance Centre (1983). *Notes on the control of human sources of gastro-intestinal infections, infestations and bacterial intoxications in the United Kingdom.* Communicable Disease Report, Supplement 1.
6. *Report of the Committee on Infectious Diseases, American Academy of Pediatrics* ('The Red Book'), (20th edn) (1986).
   To acquire this very complete guide to infectious diseases and immunizations it may be necessary to write to the American Academy, 141 Northwest Point Boulevard, PO Box 927, Elk Grove Village, Illinois 60007, USA.

Immunizations

7. *Immunization against infectious disease* (1988). DHSS.
   The recommended authority in the UK.
8. *British national formulary.* BMA/Pharmaceutical Society.
   Regularly updated and collects all vaccines into a handy section. Issued free to all doctors.

9. *Data sheet compendium.* Association of the British Pharmaceutical Industry, London.
    Updated annually, collates all the current data-sheets but not in a single section for immunizations. Issued free to all doctors. Data-sheets tend to be over-cautious with regard to vaccine recommendations.

Immunoglobulins

10. Indications and dosage for normal and special immunoglobulins. Blood Products Laboratory, Elstree, Middlesex. Unpublished. Available from PHLS.

Travel abroad

11. Dawood, R. (ed.) (1986). *Travellers' health.* Oxford University Press. A guide for the layman but also useful for doctors.
12. Walker, E. and Williams, G. (1985). *ABC of health travel,* (2nd edn). British Medical Association, London.
13. *Protect your health abroad.* Leaflet SA 35.
    Available: travel agents or DHSS Leaflets Unit, PO Box 21, Stanmore, Middx HA7 1AY. Updated annually, gives the current vaccination requirements of all countries.
14. *Vaccination requirements and health advice for international travel,* (1988). WHO, Geneva.
    Available from HMSO.

Official statistics England and Wales

15. Office of Population Censuses and Surveys: Annual Monitors

Series no.	Subject
DH2	Mortality by cause
DH3	Childhood and maternity mortality statistics
MB2	Infectious diseases

    Available in good medical libraries and for purchase from HMSO.
16. *Communicable Disease Reports.* Published weekly by the Centre for Disease Surveillance and Control (see p. 315).

Human Immunodeficiency Virus (HIV)

17. Batty, D. (ed.) (1987). *The implications of AIDS for children in care.* BAAF.
    Available from the British Agency for Adoption and Fostering, 11 Southwark Street, London SE1 1RQ.

18. The Royal College of Obstetricians and Gynaecologists. *Report of the RCOG sub-committee on problems associated with AIDS in relation to obstetrics and gynaecology.*
    Available from the RCOG, 27 Sussex Place, London NW1 4RG. A guide to practical management problems for obstetricians, midwives, and paediatricians dealing with HIV-positive babies.

19. British Paediatric Association (1988). *Report of a Working Party on AIDS in infancy and childhood.* In press.

Glossary and abbreviations

Active immunity	Immunity acquired during life by contact with an antigen.
Adrenaline	Drug used in treatment of anaphylaxis. Amongst other actions it stimulates the heart and relaxes bronchial spasm.
Agglutinins	One type of antibody.
AIDS	Acquired Immunodeficiency Syndrome
Anaphylaxis	A severe allergic reaction characterized by collapse, shock, poor pulse, sometimes with wheezing and swelling of the soft tissues.
Anicteric	No visible jaundice. Used to describe cases of hepatitis where no jaundice can be seen.
Antibody	A blood protein which is part of the body's immunity. Antibodies are immunoglobulins and some specific types are called agglutinins.
Antigen	Any substance which can cause an immune response from the body, such as stimulating the formation of antibodies.
Anuria	Urine flow having ceased.
Apyrexial	Absence of fever (temperature under 37.5°C).
ARC	AIDS-related complex. A condition preceding AIDS.
Attack rate	See Incidence rate.
Attenuated vaccine	A live vaccine which is derived from a disease-causing organism but altered to render it harmless.
Auscultation	Listening with a stethoscope (usually to the chest).
Barrier nursing	Strict nursing in hospital with an individual room, use of masks, gowns, and gloves by all entering the room; and handwashing after contact with the patient or potentially contaminated material before attending to other patients.
BCG	Bacille Calmette–Guerin. The vaccine against tuberculosis.
BNF	British National Formulary
Booster	A term meaning a subsequent vaccination to an initial course of injections, e.g. pre-school booster, tetanus booster.
Capsulated or encapsulated bacteria	A type of bacteria with a protective capsule.

Carrier	An individual infected with an organism but without symptoms and capable of infecting others.
CDSC	Centre for Disease Surveillance and Control
CMV	Cytomegalovirus
CNS	Central nervous system
Coagulase	The ability to coagulate plasma, an index of pathogenicity in Staphylococci.
Colonization	When an organism lives in or on another living creature without being invasive or causing disease.
Commensal	An organism which normally inhabits an area without causing symptoms, e.g. *Candida* is a skin commensal.
Confluent rash	Where the spots of the rash join up.
Coryza	An acutely running nose.
CRS	Congenital rubella syndrome
CSF	Cerebrospinal fluid
DHSS	Department of Health and Social Security
Discrete rash	A rash where the spots stay separate, cf. confluent rash.
DTP	Diphtheria/tetanus/pertussis combined vaccine
Dysentery	Diarrhoea with blood and pus (irrespective of the causative organism).
Dysuria	Pain on passing urine
EB, EBV	Epstein–Barr virus
ELISA	Enzyme-linked immunosorbent assay. A laboratory test used to diagnose a variety of diseases by detecting antibodies in blood and other body fluids.
Endemic	A disease that is always present in a community, e.g. malaria in India, measles in England.
Enteric precautions	Gloves should be used for touching contaminated materials. Hands must be washed after contact with the patient or potentially contaminated articles before contact with another person. Masks are unnecessary but gowns are needed where soiling is likely. Where possible an individual toilet facility should be used or care taken to clean a shared facility after use.
Enterotoxin	See Toxin.
Eosinophilia	A high level of a particular class of white blood cells, the eosinophils. Usually indicative of infestation or an allergic phenomenon.

Epidemic	A large-scale outbreak of disease.
Erythematous	Red appearance to skin.
Exotoxin	See Toxin.
Fatality rate	The frequency of deaths due to a disease amongst cases of the disease.
First-degree relations	For a person this includes their full brothers and sisters (siblings) and natural parents; not more distant relatives.
Fomites	Any inanimate object that may harbour a pathogenic organism, e.g. a soiled handkerchief.
HBV	Hepatitis B virus
HBVac	Vaccine against hepatitis B infection
Heaf test	One of the tests for immunity against TB.
Herd immunity	The level of immunity in the general population against a particular disease.
HIV	Human immunodeficiency virus. The cause of AIDS.
HMSO	Her Majesty's Stationery Office
Horizontal transmission	Transmission of infection from one person to another; not vertical (mother to child) transmission.
Host	An individual (human or other species) who is infected by an organism, with or without symptoms.
HRIG	Anti-rabies immunoglobulin
HSV	*Herpes simplex* virus
Hypergamma-globulinaemia	Raised gammaglobulin levels in the blood.
Hypoxia/hypo-xaemia	Low levels of oxygen in the blood.
im	intramuscular
Immunity	The ability of an individual to resist disease, especially infection. Can be natural, active or passive.
	Natural immunity—the non-specific immunity which depends on genetic and non-specific factors (e.g. mucus secretions and antiseptic agents in sweat) and makes different species susceptible to some organisms and resistant to others.
	Active immunity—the specific immunity acquired by natural or induced exposure, and achieved by

the immune system producing antibodies and cells which attack pathogens.

Passive immunity—specific immunity acquired by injection of a preparation of antibodies. This also refers to the placenta from mother to fetus.

Immunization	See Vaccine.
Immunoglobulins	See Antibody.
Inactivated or killed vaccine	A vaccine made of dead material. It may be the whole organism, e.g. pertussis, or a component, e.g. pneumococcus.
Incidence rate	The number of new cases of a disease occurring in a population of defined size per unit of time.
Incubation period	The time between a person encountering an organism and symptoms appearing.
Induration	A hard area of skin or tissue.
Infancy	From birth to the first birthday.
Infection	The invasion of a host and multiplication therein by an organism. This may or may not lead to symptoms (disease).
Infectious	A disease or organism that is commonly communicated from one host (human or otherwise) to another. Contrast with diseases which are due to infectious organisms but are not communicated from one human to another, e.g. urinary-tract infections.
Intradermal injection	Immunization by injection into the layers of the skin. Used for BCG and sometimes typhoid.
Intramuscular injection	Injection into the muscles.
iv	intravenous
Leukocytosis	High blood white cell count.
Leukopoenia	Low blood white cell count.
Live vaccine	A vaccine made of live bacteria or virus much altered so that it is not dangerous but can still induce immunity.
Lymphadenopathy	Lymph gland enlargement.
Lymphocyte	One of the white blood cells concerned in the body's immunity.
Lymphocytosis	Unusually high number of lymphocytes.
Mantoux test	A skin test for immunity against TB.
MIG	Anti-mumps immunoglobulin
MMR	Measles, mumps, rubella combined vaccine

MOEH	Medical Officer of Environmental Health. In some areas other medical officers fulfil similar functions.
Monovalent	A vaccine with only one component, e.g. pertussis.
Morbidity rate	The amount of illness occurring amongst a defined number of people in a unit of time.
Mortality rate	The number of deaths occurring amongst a defined number of people in a unit of time.
Named-person basis	A term used to indicate that an immunization is available for use if a doctor requests it from a supplier for a particular individual, but is not yet licensed for general use. For example, this is the case for the immunization for tick-borne encephalitis (1987).
Neonate	Baby in the first 4 weeks of life.
Oliguria	Low urine output.
Parenteral	Given by injection.
Passive immunity	See Immunity.
Pathogenic	Producing disease.
Per-nasal swab	A swab used to take a sample of the mucus in a child's pharynx. It is inserted through the nostrils and is used as a test for whooping cough.
Peri-	Around. Hence perianal (around the anus), perioral (around the mouth).
Pertussis	The medical term for whooping cough.
PHLS	Public Health Laboratory Service
Primary course	Applies to diphtheria, tetanus, pertussis, and polio, and means the first three immunizations.
Proctitis	Inflammation or infection around the anus.
Prodrome	Symptoms experienced prior to the characteristic features of a specific infectious disease.
Prophylaxis	The process of protecting an individual with an agent, e.g. a vaccine or an antibiotic.
PUO	Pyrexia of unknown origin.
Pyrexia	Fever.
Pyuria	A significant number of white blood (pus) cells in the urine.
Reactogenic	An immunization producing a reaction.
Reye's syndrome	A profound illness involving liver failure and general collapse which is frequently fatal.
Rigor	A systemic reaction involving shaking associated with high fever.
Rubella	The medical term for German measles.

sc	subcutaneous
Second- and third-degree relations	Relatives more distant than brother/sister and parents, e.g. a cousin.
Serology	Looking for antibodies in an individual's blood as evidence of infection.
Seropositive and seronegative	A person whose blood shows they have antibodies (and therefore are presumed immune) to a specific disease, either because they have been immunized or have had the infection. Seronegative means not having such antibodies.
SPA	Suprapubic aspiration (of urine)
Strain	A sub-type of a species of organism, e.g. the different strains of Staphylococcus.
Subclinical	An infection where there are no overt symptoms.
Subcutaneous	An injection under the skin but not into the deeper layers of muscle.
Teratogenic	Producing a malformation in the fetus.
Toxin	A poison produced by an infecting organism, e.g. toxin from diphtheria or tetanus.
Toxoid	An immunization prepared from a toxin by removing its poisonous qualities but retaining its vaccinating effects, e.g. tetanus toxoid which is tetanus toxin inactivated by formaldehyde
Triple vaccine	The immunization incorporating diphtheria, tetanus, and whooping cough (DPT).
Tympanic membrane	The ear-drum.
Vaccine	A suspension of attenuated live or killed micro-organisms or fractions thereof given to induce immunity and hence prevent infectious disease. Vaccination essentially means the same as immunization.
Vaccinee	An individual who is being immunized.
Vertical transmission	(For infectious disease) Mother-to-child transmission in the prenatal or perinatal period across the placenta, blood-borne, or via breast milk.
ZIG	Zoster immune globulin (anti-varicella immunoglobulin)

Index

Main entries are in **bold type**

abscess 21, 23
achondroplasia 256
acquired immunodeficiency syndrome *see*
    AIDS
acyclovir 32, 44–5, 81, 82, **286**
adenoviruses 7, 57, 126
adrenaline *inside back cover*
AIDS xviii, xxi, 33, **37–42**, 65, 154
    breast-feeding 41
    diagnosis 40
    epidemiology 37–8
    immunization 42, **257–8**
    incubation period 39
    infectivity 39–40
    management 41
    natural history 40
    precautions 41
    pregnancy 33
    risk groups 37–8
    transmission 38–9
allergy **256**
amikacin **286**
amikin 286
amodiaquine 271
amoebic dysentery 57, 63, 304
amoxil 286
amoxycillin 7, 9, 26, **286**
amoxycillin and clavulanic acid **287**
amphotericin **287**
ampicillin 10, 33, 62, 65, 67, 71, 125, **288**
anaphylaxis 182–3
    treatment *inside back cover*
antibiotics **287–304**
    endocarditis prophylaxis 260–1
    for gastrointestinal infection **62**
    for respiratory-tract infection 7
    for urinary-tract infection 26–7
aplastic crises 56
apnoea 3, 124, 149, 150
appendicitis 28, 29, 58
arthralgia 89
arthritis 23, 71, 86, 96, 122, 124, 126, 256,
    294
aspirin 44, 87
asplenia 256
asthma **256**

astrovirus 57
augmentin 287
avloclor 272
azlocillin **288**

bacillus Calmette–Guerin vaccine *see* BCG
Bacillus cereus 57
bacitracin 122
bacteraemia 22, 23, 71, 95–6, 211
banocide 292
BCG *inside front cover,* 140, 180
BCG immunization **224–9**, 269, 312
    administration 226–8
    contraindications 225
    Heaf test 226–7
    indications 225
    Mantoux test 226–7
    reactions 186, 228
Behcet's syndrome 24
benzyl benzoate 120
benzyl penicillin 8, 33, 34, 53, 96, 104, 125,
    298
birth asphyxia 256
Bordetella parapertussis 150
Bordetella pertusssis **148–51**
breast feeding 34
British Paediatric Surveillance Unit **xxi**
bronchiolitis xvi, **10–11**, 109–10
    treatment 11
brucellosis 23
burns 128

Campylobacter jejuni 57, 58, 62, 63, 155,
    279, 304
Candida albicans **132**
candidiasis 12, 40, **132–3**, 296
carbaryl 102
carbenicillin **288**
carylderm 102
cefotaxime 7, 71, **289**
ceftazidime **289**
cefuroxime **290**
cellulitis 71
cephaclor 71
cephradine 26, **290**
cerebral palsy 50, **257**

chickenpox xvi, 14, 15, 17, 21, 34, **43–5**, 154, 304
  diagnosis 44
  epidemiology 43
  incubation period 43
  infectivity 43
  management 44
  natural history 43
  pregnancy 34, 45
  transmission 43
Chlamydia psittaci 293
Chlamydia trachomatis 7, 11, 30, 31, 32, **46–7**, 67, 154, 293
  diagnosis 47
  epidemiology 46
  natural history 46
  pregnancy 32
  treatment 47
chloramphenicol 7, 10, 62, 71, 96, 145, **290**
chlorhexidine 122
chloromycetin 290
chloroquine 90, 272, 273, **291**
cholera xvii, **48–9**, 154, 282, 304
  epidemiology 48
  incubation period 48
  infectivity 48
  management 49
  natural history 48–9
  diagnosis 49
  transmission 48
cholera immunization **188–9**, 270
  administration 188–9
  contraindications 188
  indications 188
  reactions 189
chorioretinitis 137
Claforan 289
clavulanic acid 7, 71, **287**
Clostridium tetani 128
clotrimazole 112, 113, **291**
coeliac disease 29
condyloma acuminata 31, 146
congenital adrenal hyperplasia 28
congenital heart disease 11, 117, **257**
Congenital Rubella Surveillance Scheme 118
conjunctivitis 46, 47, 66, 67
constipation 144
convulsions 4, 69, 82, 88, 150
corticosteroids **258**
Corynebacterium diphtheriae **52**
coryza 3, **6–7**, 43, 55, 92, 116
co-trimoxazole 26, 49, 62, 71, **292**
cough 11, 84, 92, 144, 149
coxsackie virus 73
Crohn's disease 24, 29

crotamiton 120
croup **9–10**, 52
  treatment 10
crying 4
Cryptosporidium 57, 155
crystapen 298
cyanosis 11
cyanotic attacks 150
cystic fibrosis 29, 84, 122, 289, 295, 297
  immunization **257**
cytomegalic inclusion disease 50
cytomegalovirus (CMV) 3, 32, **50–51**, 154
  diagnosis 51
  epidemiology 50
  incubation period 50
  infectivity 50
  management 51
  natural history 50
  pregnancy 32, 50
  transmission 50

daktarin 296
deafness 3, 9, 100, 117
dehydration 48, **58–61**
  hypernatraemic 60
  isotonic 60
deltoid muscle 178
derbac 102
dermatitis herpetiformis 14, 16, 17
diabetes mellitus 257
diagnosis of infection **153–9**
diarrhoea 29, 40, 48, 57, 58, 60, 86, 144
diethyl toluamide (DEET) 271
diethylcarbamazine **292**
dioralyte 60
diphtheria xvi, xvii, **52–4**, 65, 154, 279, 280, 304
  antitoxin 53
  diagnosis 53
  epidemiology 52
  incubation period 52
  infectivity 52
  management 53
  natural history 52
  transmission 52
diphtheria immunization **190–1**, 269
  administration 191
  contraindications 191
  indications 190
  reactions 191
Down's syndrome **257**
DTP immunization *inside front cover,* 312
  reactions 184–5

econazole 113
ectodermal dysplasia 24
eczema herpeticum 16, 17, 21, 82, 286
empyema 71, 121
encephalitis 28, 44, 80, 82, 84, 117, 150
encephalopathy 40, 92, 93
endocarditis 23, 96, 126, 298
endocarditis prophylaxis **260–1**
endocervicitis 67
endocrine disorders 257
Entamoeba histolytica 62
Enterobius vermicularis 130
enteroviral infections 16, 20, 32
enterovirus 57, 105
epiglottitis **9–10**, 70, 290
    treatment 10
Epstein–Barr virus (EBV) 7, 8, **64**, 126
erysipelas 298
erythema infectiosum 16, 18, **55–6**, 304
    diagnosis 56
    epidemiology 55
    incubation period 55
    infectivity 55
    natural history 55–6
    transmission 55
    treatment 56
erythema toxicum 14
erythromycin 47, 62, 67, 104, 150, **293**
erythroped 293
Escherichia coli 26, 57, 63, 68, 155, 279, 304
ethambutol 142, **293**
eurax 120
European tick-borne encephalitis 277
exanthem subitum 15, 16, 18, 20, **114**
exclusion periods **305–11**

failure to thrive 40
Fansidar 271
febrile convulsions 5, 257
fever 3, 9, 12, **22–4**, 43, 52, 55, 64, 73, 82,
    84, 85, 88, 92, 96, 99, 106, 107, 140,
    144, 152
fifth disease 16, 18, **55–6**, 304
    diagnosis 56
    epidemiology 55
    incubation period 55
    infectivity 55
    natural history 55–6
    transmission 55
    treatment 56
flagyl 296
floppiness 3
floxapen 294
flucloxacillin 122, **294**

folinic acid 34
food poisoning 122
fucidin 294
fungizone 287
fusidic acid 122, **294**

gastroenteritis 22
gastrointestinal infections **57–63**
    diagnosis 58
    epidemiology 57
    management 58
    natural history 57
    transmission 57
gastrointestinal tuberculosis 140
genital warts 30
gentamicin **295**
genticin 295
Giardia lamblia see giardiasis
giardiasis 57, 62, 63, 155, 280, 296, 304
gingivostomatitis 82
glandular fever 8, 16, 18, 22, 23, **64–5**, 87,
        155, 306
    diagnosis 65
    epidemiology 64
    incubation period 64
    infectivity 64
    natural history 64–5
    transmission 64
    treatment 65
glomerulonephritis 8, 125, 126
glucose electrolyte mixture 60
gonococcal infections 30, 31, 33, **66–7**, 156,
        298
    diagnosis 67
    epidemiology 66
    incubation period 66
    infectivity 66
    natural history 66–7
    pregnancy 33
    transmission 66
    treatment 67
Gram stain 14, 67
griseofulvin 112, **295**
growth hormone deficiency 257

haematuria 68
haemolytic anaemia 69
haemolytic uraemia syndrome xviii, xxi, 29,
        68–9
    epidemiology 68
    natural history 68–9
    treatment 69
haemophilia 257

Haemophilus influenzae 7, 9, 10, 11, 12,
   70–1, 155, 290, 301
   diagnosis 71
   epidemiology 70
   incubation period 70
   meningitis xvii
   natural history 70–1
   transmission 70
   treatment 71
haemorrhagic shock encephalopathy syndrome xxi
hand, foot, and mouth disease 14, 17, 21,
   73–4, 306
   diagnosis 73
   epidemiology 73
   incubation period 73
   infectivity 73
   management 73
   natural history 73
   transmission 73
head louse 101, 308
headache 9, 64, 75, 84, 99
Heaf test 141, **226–7**, 312
hepatitis 22, 23, 28, 44, 50, 51, 75–9, 78, 80,
   143
hepatitis A **75–6**, 155, **274–5**, 279, 280, 306
   diagnosis 76
   epidemiology 75
   incubation period 75
   infectivity 75
   management 76
   natural history 75–6
   transmission 75
hepatitis B, 32, **77–9**, 155, 306
   diagnosis 78–9
   epidemiology 77
   incubation period 78
   infectivity 78
   managment 79
   natural history 78
   pregnancy 32, 77
hepatitis B immunization 79, **192–6**
   active 192
   administration 194–5
   contraindications 194
   high risk group 193–4
   in newborn 193
   passive 192
   reactions 195
hepatomegaly 144
hepatosplenomegaly 40, 137
herpes simplex xvi, 16, 17, 21, 30, 31, 32,
   80–2, 155, 286, 306
   in childhood 81–2
   diagnosis 82

   epidemiology 81
   incubation period 82
   infectivity 82
   natural history 82
   transmission 82
   treatment 82
   in newborn xviii, xxi, 80–1
   diagnosis 81
   epidemiology 80
   infectivity 80
   management 81
   natural history 80
   transmission 80
   in pregnancy 32, 81
herpes zoster 16, **44**, 154
hexachlorophane 122
hiatus hernia 28
Hirschsprung's disease 28
histiocytosis 24
HIV infection 33, **37–42**, 65, 142, 154
hookworm 302
human immunodeficiency virus (HIV)
   infection 33, **37–42**, 65, 142, 154
   immunization **257–8**
human normal immunoglobulin (HNIG) **76**,
   274–5
human papilloma virus (HPV) 31, **146**
human rabies immunoglobulin (HRIG) **276**
hydrocephalus 137, **258**
hypertension 69
hypoxia 149

idiopathic respiratory distress syndrome 124
idiopathic thrombocytopaenic purpura
   (ITP) 20
IHAH *see* isoniazid
immunization
   accelerated schedules 313–14
   BCG *inside back cover* **224–9**, 269
   catch-up schedules **313–14**
   cholera **188–9**, 270
   consent 173
   contraindications 164–6
   diphtheria xx, **190–1**, 269
   diphtheria/tetanus/pertussis *inside back
      cover*, 54
   dosages 179
   European tick-borne encephalitis 277
   Heaf *inside back cover*
   Health Visitors 172–3
   hepatitis B **192–6**
   immunodeficiency 166
   influenza **197–9**
   injection site 178

intradermal injection 180–1
intramuscular injection 179–80
malaria **270–4**
Mantoux *inside back cover*
measles xx, **205**, 269, *inside back cover*
MMR 100, **200–4**, *inside back cover*
mumps **206**, *inside back cover*
parental counselling 174–5
pertussis xx, **207–10**
pneumococcal **211–12**
polio xx, **213–16**, 268, *inside back cover*
polio (IPV) **216**
polio (OPV) **213–15**
rabies **275–7**
reactions 182–7
record 181
rubella **217–20**, *inside back cover*
subcutaneous injection 179–80
tetanus xx, **221–3**, 269
tuberculosis **224–9**
typhoid **230–1**, 269–70
yellow card 184
yellow fever **232–3**, 270
immunization checklist, *inside front cover*,
    177–81
immunization myths 167
immunization questions and answers **239–55**
    after injury 254
    allergies 248, 249
    asthma 248, 249
    babies on antibiotics 244
    breast-feeding 241
    cerebral damage 240
    cerebral palsy 247
    congenital heart disease 247
    cystic fibrosis 247
    developmental delay 246
    eczema 248, 249
    family epilepsy 248
    hay fever 248, 249
    hydrocephalus 247
    interrupted immunization course 249
    neurological disease 246
    pregnancy 251
    premature babies 241
    previous reactions 244
    previous fits or febrile convulsions 245
    spina bifida 247
    steroids 244
    unwell babies 241–3
immunization schedule, *inside back cover*
immunization targets xix
    diphtheria xix
    measles/mumps/rubella xix
    pertussis xix

polio xix
rubella xix
tetanus xix
immunization technique 179–81
immunization uptake xx
immunodeficiency 12, 214, 218, 225, **258**
immunodepressed **258**
immunoglobulin preparations **234–6**
    chickenpox-zoster immune globulin
        (ZIG) 44, 45, 235
    hepatitis A **76**, 235
    hepatitis B 235
    measles 235
    mumps 235
    normal 234
    tetanus 236
impetigo 16, 17, 21, 125, 306
incubation periods **305–11**
infectious mononucleosis 8, 16, 18, 22, 23,
        64–5, 87, 155, 306
    diagnosis 65
    epidemiology 64
    incubation period 64
    infectivity 64
    natural history 64–5
    transmission 64
    treatment 65
influenza **83–4**, 156, 306
    diagnosis 84
    epidemiology 83
    incubation period 83
    infectivity 83
    natural history 84
    transmission 83
    treatment 84
influenza immunization 84, **197–9**
    administration 198
    contraindications 198
    indications 197–8
    reactions 198
influenza viruses **83**
insect bites 16, 17, 21
intracranial calcification 137
intussusception 28, 58
irritability 3
isoniazid 33, 142, **295**

jaundice xvii, 50, 75, 76, 78, 89, 137, 152
juvenile rheumatoid arthritis 87, 259

kaolin 59
Kaposi's varicelliform eruption 82
Kawasaki disease xviii, xxi, 16, 19, 23, 29,
        85–7

Kawasaki disease (*cont.*)
  diagnosis 86
  epidemiology 85
  management 87
  natural history 85
  transmission 85
Klebsiella pneumoniae 84
Koplik's spots 92

laryngotracheobronchitis **9**, 52
Lassa fever 280
legionella 293
leucocytosis 65
leukaemia 20, 24, 258
leukopenia 65
lice **101–2**, 308
Listeria monocytogenes infection 23, 33
listeriosis 23, 33
loperamide 59
lymphadenopathy 40, 64, 86, 117
lymphoblastic leukaemia 65
lymphomas 24

malaria xvii, 20, 22, 23, **88–90**, 156, 270–5,
    280, 282, 301, 306
  diagnosis 89
  epidemiology 88
  incubation period 88
  management 89
  natural history 88–9
  prophylaxis 270–5
  transmission 88
malathion 102
malignancy and immunization 258–9
maloprim 272, 273
malrotation 28
Mantoux test 141, 180, **226–7**, 312
measles xvi, xvii, 15, 16, 18, 28, 33, 87,
    91–4, 156, 306
  diagnosis 93
  epidemiology 91
  immune globulin 93
  immunosuppression 93
  incubation period 91
  infectivity 91
  management 93
  natural history 92–3
  pregnancy 33
  transmission 91
measles immunization 93, **200–5**, 269
  reactions 185–6
measles virus **91**
measles/mumps/rubella immunization *see*
    MMR

mebendazole 131, **295**
meningitis xvi, xvii, 4, 5, 22, 28, 58, 65, 70,
    86, 96, 104, 106, 122, 124, 141, 211,
    277, 279, 280, 287, 288, 289, 290, 298
  immunization 259
  viral xvii
meningo-encephalitis 99–100
meningococcaemia 96
meningococcal infection 5, 16, 19, **95–7**, 156,
    298, 306
  diagnosis 96
  epidemiology 95
  immunization 97
  incubation period 95
  management 96–7
  meningitis xvii
  natural history 95–6
  transmission 95
metronidazole 62, **296**
miconazole 133, **296**
microcephaly 3, 50
Microsporum 111
migraine 28
miliary TB 140
MMR immunization *inside front cover*,
    200–4, 312
  administration 202
  contraindications 202
  indications 201–2
  reactions 185–6, 203
Molluscum contagiosum 16, 17, **98**, 156, 306
  diagnosis 98
  epidemiology 98
  management 98
  natural history 98
  transmission 98
Monospot tests 65
monosulfiram 120
mucocutaneous lymph node syndrome
    (MCNLS) xviii, xxi, 16, 19, 23, 29,
    85–7
  diagnosis 86
  epidemiology 85
  management 87
  natural history 85
  transmission 85
mumps xvi, 33, **99–100**, 156, 308
  diagnosis 100
  epidemiology 99
  incubation period 99
  infectivity 99
  management 99
  natural history 99–100
  pregnancy 33, 99
  transmission 99

mumps immunization **206**
Munchausen by proxy syndrome 24
myambutol 293
Mycobacterium tuberculosis 7, 33, **139**
Mycoplasma pneumoniae 7, 11
myocarditis 84

naseptin 122
nasopharyngitis 52
National Immunization Schedule 312–13
Neisseria gonorrhoea 30, 31, 33, **66**, 156, 298
Neisseria meningitidis **95**, 301
neomycin 122
neonatal urticaria 14
nephrotic syndrome 103, 259
netillin 297
netilmicin **297**
neurodegenerative disorders 24
nitrofurantoin 27, **297**
nits **101–2**, 308
    diagnosis 101–2
    epidemiology 101
    infectivity 101
    management 102
    natural history 101
    transmission 101
nivaquine 272
non-gonococcal urethritis 46
notifiable diseases 284
nystatin 133, **297**

oesophageal stricture 28
oliguria 68
ophthalmia neonatorum xvii, 46, 66, 285
optic neuritis 143
osteomyelitis 23, 122, 124, 294
otitis media 4, **8–9**, 22, 58, 70, 84, 92, 104, 124, 126, 286, 288
    treatment 9
otrivine 7

paludrine 272
pancreatitis 44, 100
paracetamol 7, 209
para-influenzae viruses 7
paratyphoid 282
paronychia 121
parotid gland 99
parotitis 100
parvovirus B19 55
Paul Bunnell tests 65

Pediculus humanus capitis **101**, 308
pelvic inflammatory disease 67
pemphigus 14
Penbritin 288
penicillin 7
pencillin G **298**
penicillin V 8, **299**
per-nasal swab 150
pertussis xvi, xvii, **148–51**, 157, 310
    diagnosis 150
    epidemiology 148
    incubation period 148
    infectivity 148
    management 150–1
    natural history 149
    transmission 148
pertussis immunization **207–10**
    administration 208
    cerebral irritation 209
    contraindications 208
    convulsions 209
    family members with epilepsy 209
    homeopathic vaccine 210
    indications 207
    reactions 208–9
petechiae 126
pharyngitis 8, 67, 126
phenoxymethylpenicillin (penicillin V) 8, 104, **299**
photophobia 92
piperacillin **299**
piperazine 131, **299**
Pipril 299
pityriasis rosea 19, 20
pivampicillin **300**
Plasmodium falciparum **88**
pneumococcal immunization 104, **211–12**
    administration 212
    contraindications 212
    indications 211
    reactions 212
pneumococcal infections xvii, **103–4**, 298
    diagnosis 104
    epidemiology 103
    incubation period 103
    infectivity 103
    natural history 103–4
    transmission 103
    treatment 104
pneumococcus (*S. pneumoniae*) 9, **103**, 156
pneumocystis pneumonia 292
Pneumocystis carinii 12, 292
pneumonia xvi, 5, **11–12**, 22, 25, 44, 46, 51, 65, 71, 84, 86, 92, 96, 103, 121, 124, 150, 211, 286, 288, 298

polio *see* poliomyelitis
polio immunization 268, 312
  reactions 186
polio (IPV) immunization 216
polio (OPV) immunization **213–15**
  administration 214
  contraindications 214
  indications 213
  reactions 215
polio virus 105
poliomyelitis *inside front cover* xvi, xvii,
  105–6, 156, 279, 280, 308
  epidemiology 105
  incubation period 105
  infectivity 105
  management 106
  natural history 106
  transmission 105
polymixin 122
pondocillin 300
post-enteritis syndrome 60
poxvirus 98
pregnancy
  AIDS infection 33
  chickenpox infection 34
  Chlamydia trachomatis infection 32
  cytomegalovirus infection 32
  enterovirus infection 32
  hepatitis B infection 32
  herpes simplex virus infection 32
  human immunodeficiency virus
    infection 33
  immunization **259**
  infections and breast-feeding 34
  Listeria monocytogenes infection 33
  measles infection 33
  mumps infection 33
  Mycobacterium tuberculosis infection 33
  Neisseria gonorrhoea infection 33
  rubella infection 33
  Streptococcus agalactiae infection 33
  syphilis infection 34
  Toxoplasma gondii infection 34
  Treponema pallidum infection 34
  varicella infection 34
prematurity 259
prioderm 102
pripsen 299
probenecid 298
procaine penicillin 67, **298**
proctitis 67
proguanil 272, 273
proteinuria 68
pruritus 101, 119, 130
Pseudomonas aeruginosa 289, 299

Public Health Laboratories **315**
PUO **23–4**
purpura 96
pyelonephritis 26
pyloric stenosis 28
pyopen 288
pyrazinamide 142, **300**
pyrexia of unknown origin **23–4**
pyrexia 3
pyrimethamine 34, 271, 272
pyuria 26, 86

quinine **300**

rabies **107–8**, 275–7, 280, 281, 282
  diagnosis 107–8
  epidemiology 107
  incubation period 107
  natural history 107
  transmission 107
rabies immunization **275–7**
rash 4, 43, 55, 65, 73, 78, 86, 91–2, 96, 116,
  126, 144
rashes **13–21**
  haemorraghic 14
  maculopapular 14
  punctiform 14
  vesicular 14
rehidrat 60
relapsing fever 23
renal failure 68
respiratory infections **6–12**
  antibiotics for 7
respiratory syncytial virus (RSV) infection 3,
  7, 10, 11, **109–10**, 157
  diagnosis 110
  epidemiology 109
  incubation period 109
  infectivity 109
  management 110
  natural history 109–10
  transmission 109
Reye's syndrome xxi, 28, 44
rheumatic fever 8, 125, 299
rhinoviruses 7, 8
ribavirin 110
rifampicin 71, 96, 142, **301**
ringworm **111–13**, 295, 308
  diagnosis 112
  epidemiology 111
  incubation period 111
  infectivity 111

management 112–13
natural history 111–12
of body 112
of foot 112, 113
of nail 112, 113
of scalp 111, 112
transmission 111
roseola infantum 15, 16, 18, 20, 87, **114**
diagnosis 114
epidemiology 114
management 114
natural history 114
transmission 114
rotavirus 57, 63, 155, 308
roundworm 302
rubella *inside front cover*, xvi, xviii, 3, 15,
19, 20, 33, **115–18**, 157, 308
congenital infection 117
Congenital Rubella Surveillance
Scheme 118
diagnosis 117
epidemiology 115
incubation period 115
infection of child and adult 116
infectivity 115
management 117–18
natural history 116–17
pregnancy 33, 117
pregnancy and immunization 117
transmission 115
rubella immunization 117, 118, 217–20, 312
administration 218
arthritis 219
contraindications 218
immigrant women 220
indications 217
postnatal 220
reactions 218–19, 186

Salmonella typhi 62, **144**
Salmonella see salmonellosis
salmonellosis 57, 63, 155, 279, 292
sarcoma 24
Sarcoptes scabiei 119
scabies 21, **119–20**, 308
diagnosis 120
epidemiology 119
incubation period 119
infectivity 119
management 120
natural history 119–20
transmission 119
scalded skin syndrome 122
scarlet fever xvii, 15, 19, 20, 87, 124, **126**

sciatic nerve 178
securopen 288
sensorineural deafness 51
septicaemia xvi, 104, 121, 126
sexual abuse 30, 47, 66, 67, 82, 98, 147
microbiological tests **30–1**
sexually transmitted disease **30–1**
diagnosis **30–1**
Shigella see shigellosis
shigellosis 57, 58, 62, 63, 155, 279, 308
shingles **44**, 82
sickle-cell anaemia 103
sickle-cell disease 259
sinusitis 23
sixth disease 18
slapped cheeks syndrome 16, 18, **55–6**, 304
spectinomycin 67
spiramycin 34
spleen 211
splenectomy 103, **256**, 259, 299
splenomegaly 65, 89, 144
staphylococcal infections **121–3**
diagnosis 122
epidemiology 121
incubation period 121
infectivity 121
natural history 121–2
prevention 122
transmission 121
treatment 122
Staphylococcus aureus 11, 12, 57, 84, **121**,
157, 287
Staphylococcus epidermidis 121
steroids 260
streptococcal infections **124–7**
streptococcal tonsillitis 65, 126
Streptococcus agalactiae 3, 33, **124–5**
diagnosis 125
epidemiology 124
incubation period 124
natural history 124–5
pregnancy 33, 124
transmission 124
treatment 125
Streptococcus pneumoniae 11, 12, **103–4**,
211
Streptococcus pyogenes 7, 8, 9, **125–7**
diagnosis 126
epidemiology 125
incubation period 125
infectivity 125
natural history 126
scarlet fever 126
transmission 125
treatment 126–7

streptomycin 142, **302**
stridor 9, 84
strongyloides 302
subacute sclerosing panencephalitis (SSPE)
    xviii, xxi, 92
sudden infant death syndrome xvi, 109
sulphadiazine 34
suprapubic aspiration of urine 26, 159
syphilis 34, 67
systemic juvenile rheumatoid arthritis 24
systemic lupus erythematosus 24

tachypnoea 3, 11, 12, 110
tetanus xvii, **128–9**, 157, 308
    diagnosis 129
    epidemiology 128
    immune globulin 129
    incubation period 128
    natural history 128
    transmission 128
    treatment 129
tetanus immunization **221–3**, 269
    administration 222
    contraindications 222
    indications 221
    reactions 222
tetmosol 120
tetracycline 32, 47, 49
thalassaemia 260
thermometer 4
thiabendazole **302**
threadworms **130–1**, 302
    diagnosis 130
    epidemiology 130
    natural history 130
    transmission 130
    treatment 131
thrombocytopaenia 50, 69, 137
thrombocytosis 86
thrush 12, 40, **132–3**, 157, 296–7
    diagnosis 132–3
    epidemiology 132
    natural history 132
    transmission 132
    treatment 133
tincture of iodine 267
tinea **111–13**, 157, 291
Tinea pedis see tinea
toddler diarrhoea 29
tonsillitis 8, 22, 25, 52, 64, 65, 126, 298
    treatment 8
toxic shock syndrome 122
Toxocara canis see toxocariasis
Toxocara catis see toxocariasis

toxocariasis **134–5**
    diagnosis 134
    epidemiology 134
    infectivity 134
    management 135
    natural history 134
    prevention 135
    transmission 134
Toxoplasma gondii see toxoplasmosis
toxoplasmosis 34, **136–8**
    diagnosis 137
    epidemiology 136
    incubation period 136
    infectivity 137
    management 138
    natural history 137
    pregnancy 34, 136–7
    prevention 138
    transmisson 136
trachoma 46
transverse myelitis 65
Treponema pallidum **34**
trichomonas vaginalis 31
Trichophyton 111
trimethoprin 26, 62, **302**
triple vaccine 190, 207, 221
tuberculin test 141, 142, 225
tuberculosis xvi, xvii, 12, 23, **139–43**, 157,
    279, 280, 293, 295, 301, 308
    diagnosis of pulmonary TB 140–1
    diagnosis of TB meningitis 141
    epidemiology 139
    incubation period 139
    infectivity 139
    management during infancy 141–2
    management during childhood 142–3
    management during pregnancy 33
    management of pulmonary TB 142–3
    management of miliary TB 143
    management of meningitis 143
    natural history 140
    transmission 139
tuberculosis immunization **224–9**
tuberculous meningitis xvii, 143, 295, 300,
    302
typhoid xvii, 23, 63, 157, 280, 282, 290, 292
typhoid fever **144–5**, 308
    diagnosis 145
    epidemiology 144
    incubation period 144
    infectivity 144
    management 145
    natural history 144
    transmission 144
typhoid immunization **230–1**, 269–70

administration 231
contraindications 230
indications 230
reactions 231

ulcerative colitis 24, 29, 58
ureteric reflux 27
urinary-tract infection 4, 5, 22, 23, **25–7**, 28, 29, 58, 292, 297, 302
diagnosis 25–7
treatment 26–7
urobilinogen 76

vaccination *see* immunization
vaccine
disposal 170–1
manufacturers and suppliers 319–30
storage 169–70
transport 169–70
vaginitis 66
varicella xvi, 14, 15, 17, 21, 34, **43–5**, 154, 286, 304
diagnosis 44
epidemiology 43
incubation period 43
infectivity 43
management 44
natural history 43
neonatal 45
pregnancy 34, 45
transmission 43
varicella embryopathy 44
velosef 290
vermox 295
verotoxin 68
verrucae **146–7**, 308
diagnosis 147
epidemiology 146
incubation period 146
infectivity 146
management 147
natural history 146
transmission 146
Vibrio cholerae **48**, 57, 62

viral haemorraghic fever 282
visceral larva migrans **134–5**, 302
volvulus 28
vomiting **28**, 48, 57, 58, 60, 75, 149

warts 31, **146–7**, 157, 308
diagnosis 147
epidemiology 146
incubation period 146
infectivity 146
management 147
natural history 146
transmission 146
water sterilization 266–7
wheezing 11
whipworm 302
whooping cough xvi, xvii, **148–51**, 157, 310
diagnosis 150
epidemiology 148
incubation period 148
infectivity 148
management 150–1
natural history 149
transmission 148
wound infections, 121

yellow fever **152**, 157, 280, 282
diagnosis 152
epidemiology 152
incubation period 152
natural history 152
transmission 152
yellow fever immunization **232–3**, 270
contraindications 232
indications 232
reactions 233
Yersinia enterocolitica 57, 58

zinacef 290
zinamide 300
zoster 82
zoster immunoglobulin 34, 44–5
zovirax 286

Managing anaphylaxis

1. Lie the patient down on a flat surface in the left lateral position and maintain airway.

2. Check central pulses (neck, femoral).
   (a) If pulses are STRONG, summon medical help but no '999' call needed as this is probably a faint.
   (b) If pulses are WEAK, proceed with subcutaneous or intramuscular adrenaline, apply oxygen (if available) and summon immediate assistance—call for a doctor and if necessary make an emergency call. Drug dosage intramuscular adrenaline **1:1000**.

Less than 1 year	0.05 ml im
1st to 2nd birthday	0.1 ml im
2nd to 3rd birthday	0.2 ml im
3rd to 5th birthday	0.3 ml im
5th to 6th birthday	0.4 ml im
After 6th birthday	0.5 ml im

3. If there is no improvement in the patient's condition in 10 minutes, repeat the same dose of intramuscular adrenaline.

4. If medical assistance has not arrived after 30 minutes and the patient's condition gives rise for concern, repeat the same dose of intramuscular adrenaline.

5. **A maximum of 3 doses** of adrenaline 1 : 1000 may be given.